Arthritis and the Gut Connection

A SELF-HELP SUCCESS STORY

MARY ANNE LILLY

Australia

Mary Anne Lilly C/- Intertype Publish and Print
Unit 45, 125 Highbury Road
BURWOOD VIC 3125
www.intertype.com.au

Ordering Information:
Quantity sales. Special discounts are available on quantity purchases by corporations, associations, and others. For details, contact the "Special Sales Department" at the address above.

The publisher's catalogue record is as follows:

Lilly, Mary Anne. Arthritis and the gut connection: a self-help success story

1. Lilly, Mary Anne – Health and healing
2. Lilly, Mary Anne – Arthritis
3. Gut infection – Australia – Autobiography – Memoir
4. Autoimmune diseases – Rheumatoid arthritis – Australia
5. Integrative Medicine – Gut microbiome – Treatment – Australia
6. Functional Medicine – Gut dysbiosis – Treatment – Australia
7. Diagnosis – Prognosis – Australia – Case study

Arthritis and the Gut Connection/ Mary Anne Lilly. —1st ed.
ISBN 978-0-6455754-6-0

Contents

EPIGRAM

"But I'm just a sample of one," I said to Dr Clay Golledge, a world-renowned clinical microbiologist.

"Yes," he replied, "but you are an important sample".

DEDICATION

From the moment we first met in September 2011 there were no more put-downs. There were also no dire predictions of how a dreaded, chronic arthritic condition was going to unfold. He showed respect for the efforts I'd made to inform myself. My investigations weren't disparaged or dismissed in an off-hand manner. By contrast I was complimented with a generous remark. Dr Hira Singh simply said:

"I am very impressed. If others did this, they too could get better."

ACKNOWLEDGEMENTS

I'm greatly indebted to my dear husband Peter as without his unwavering support this story would never have been completed.

Gratitude to Grandpa Dick who encouraged me by saying:

"Mary Anne, keep records; continue your investigations. I admire your determination."

Disclaimer

In writing this memoir, I have relied upon personal journals, medical records, my recollections and information gained from reputable sources; viz. my doctors & specialists, and scientific & medical texts and websites. Knowledge has been drawn from modern medicine, as well as traditional medicines and lifestyles.

I have changed a few of the names and identifying details to preserve anonymity. In some cases, where individuals have agreed, I have retained real names and details.

Readers must be aware that everyone is different. Even though I have successfully pushed my arthritis into remission, my holistic treatment program may not work for others. Opinions and advice should be obtained from qualified health professionals.

FOREWORD

The Biomedical model on which the practice of Allopathic Medicine is based has been the dominant paradigm of our times. More recently, the Bio-Psycho-Social-Environmental model has provided us with a broader and more holistic understanding of the interplay between genetics, personal lifestyle factors, emotional and mental states, and their impact on our health. Evidence is emerging clarifying the complex relationships between biological agents (viruses, bacteria, fungi) and the human host.

Interest in the gut microbiome especially is starting to reveal its important role in maintaining homeostasis. At the same time, the role of stress is being acknowledged as a contributing background factor which disrupts the delicate balance of key hormones and neurotransmitters as well as the gut microbiome. Antigenic material from biological pathogens triggers the formation of antigen-antibody complexes resulting in inflammation – now recognized as the key pathway leading to dysfunction in multiple organ systems in the body.

The author of this personal documentary is to be commended for her relentless search for answers to her health problems. Not satisfied with a merely reductionist explanation, she researched and found the complex web of interactions in the context of her life. This new understanding resulted in a deeper level of healing for her.

I hope that this personal testimony will encourage many others to look beyond the limited perspective of a disempowering disease-label and transform their health crisis into an opportunity for growth.

Dr Hira Singh MB BS FRACGP ...Integrative Medicine Practitioner

PROLOGUE

The first indications that all was not well were subtle signals and skin changes.

Symptoms of my unhealthy gut made themselves evident on my face and elsewhere before my joints became affected. These changes marked the start of my arthritis story – initially a confusing and perplexing experience. It's what prompted me **to write the book that I would've liked to have found alongside Jenkins and Jenner's self-help arthritis guides in the Nedlands library.**

When in 2014 Dr Karen Hitchcock published an article in *The Monthly,* an Australian journal, she provided me with all the incentive I needed to tell my story. She stated that:

"Changes in medical paradigms are slow and fraught. A real paradigm change in medicine starts as a story that may one day be proven true."

It is my hope that if others achieve the same success that I have, this may come to fruition.

Chapter 1 INTRODUCTION

It's 2021 as I start to put pen to paper. This date is significant. During the last decade the medical establishment has done an about-turn regarding their explanation of osteoarthritis and has modified its treatment of some patients with rheumatoid arthritis. I was caught up in this significant shift in understanding. My case piqued the interest of doctors who were aware of the recent advances being made by medical researchers. I became an enthusiastic LAB RAT.

This is my story of how I overcame arthritis by:

- Informing myself
- Sourcing effective treatment
- Making critical lifestyle changes
- Fully recovering
- Remaining symptom free

Chapter 2 EARLY WARNING SIGNS (2010)

My first acute attack in 2010, plus troubling, unpleasant sensations

When I suffered my first excruciatingly painful encounter with arthritis, the experience was frightful, too frightful to ignore. I didn't hesitate before making a doctor's appointment first thing the following morning. It was strange that the episode occurred in the middle of the night. Nothing that I could think of had prompted the onset. Yet the pain was so sharp and penetrating, it shocked me out of a deep sleep. The intense discomfort emanating from within the right side of my groin was so severe that I flung back my bedclothes and swung my leg upwards. Next thing I found myself swinging my leg up and down, then to and fro. The pain was crippling.

The pain was nothing like anything I'd ever experienced before. I couldn't even manage to stumble to the bathroom for an aspirin. Yet it was extraordinary that the discomfort vanished in the night as suddenly as it had appeared.

This first encounter hit me like a bolt out of the blue. Besides the frightening experience, it distressed me that initially it was a struggle to find medical help. What I needed was an explanation for the crippling, but short-lived pain. Instead I was met with cryptic responses that simply added to my anxiety and left me confused. Worse still I got the impression that perhaps those I sought help from thought I was unhinged.

The GP I consulted merely studied my gait (ease of walking) and then firmly informed me that I had tendonitis. This for me simply didn't ring true, especially as the discomfort started to spread down my right leg. My once, blissfully deep sleep became broken. This time it was throbbing in my knee that woke me and prevented me from getting back to sleep. I tried smothering the troubling sensation by lying on my stomach and pressing my right knee as hard as I could into the mattress. It was to no avail. I had to resort to aspirin, but at least I was able to get to the bathroom.

My dear husband of many years became alarmed and thought the throbbing simply shouldn't be dismissed. As I'm also not one to ignore ominous signs, I landed up knocking repeatedly on the GP's door. There were still no answers; no further explanations. I wondered whether there was a physical cause. I wondered whether my love of gardening, or my long, brisk walks had triggered the "tendonitis".

However, my husband and I thought it odd that only my right-hand side was affected. We considered other possibilities. Could it be the mobile phone I always kept in my right pocket? Was it the daily habit of mine to quickly swish a towel over the bathroom floor using my right leg as a broomstick; was this lazy method I used to keep the navy tiles looking half decent to blame? After all it seemed obvious that swinging my leg around like that might not be doing my right hip, or to be precise the ligaments around the joint, much good.

In desperation I turned to the internet for help. Maybe someone else had experienced something similar? I found a helpful medical website from the USA which provided an instant diagnostic service for a moderate fee.

All I had to do was ask the doctor on the other end of the line whether he recognised my symptoms. By now I had quite a list; viz.

1. An excruciating acute attack, that appeared suddenly out of the blue in the middle of the night.
2. Uncomfortable pulling sensations on the right side of my groin when I walked.

3. More recent, nightly throbbing in my right knee.

It didn't take long before I received helpful feedback from a doctor on the other side of the world who provided me with a very plausible explanation:

"You have a cyst in your inner-hip socket. You need to be referred to an orthopaedic surgeon to have a sample of synovial fluid collected from your joint (a procedure called Joint Aspiration). This will help determine the underlying cause of the cyst and facilitate treatment."

My anxiety was heightened by the statement:

"If left untreated, this condition can cause permanent, long-term, joint damage".

This doctor in the USA then hinted at a possible explanation:

"There's a major association between bowel infections and arthritis".

Now I had serious doubts about the "tendonitis" diagnosis.

Unintentional beneficial antibiotic treatment

If the GP wasn't going to take me seriously, I needed to enlist my husband's support. He found time in his busy work schedule to accompany me to my next doctor's appointment. This brought about a noticeable change in the doctor's attitude.

However, the change that occurred in the surgery wasn't altogether to my liking. I found myself relegated to "patient status". I was thrust to one side and referred to in the 3rd person.

The good thing was that the GP appeared to sit up and take more notice. He requested a range of blood tests, together with a urine test. When the test results came back I think the three of us were all a bit startled to discover I had a severe bladder infection. Macrodantin was immediately prescribed.

It turned out that the bladder infection had been serendipitous, as the antibiotic treatment brought me great relief. Not only was the bladder infection quickly cleared, but the throbbing in my right leg ceased. This to my mind was extraordinary. Instead of relaxing into complacency, I continued to wonder to myself:

What had caused the troublesome, painful sensations in my right leg? Why had they now suddenly vanished?

Naturally I again questioned the GP, to hopefully find out what had occurred. He couldn't tell me much, but simply stated that:

"Sometimes when doctors treat one condition, they unintentionally treat something else as well."

What I found particularly encouraging is that he noted in my medical records that I was now "walking freely."

Chapter 3 ARTHRITIS DIAGNOSED (Apr 2011)

A grim prognosis

As I am a qualified librarian with a Masters Degree obtained by research, I was well equipped to further my investigations. To my mind the effectiveness of the antibiotic macrodantin suggested an infection had been the cause of my throbbing leg. The question now in the forefront of my mind became:

"What was the source of the infection?"

I continued to inform myself using the internet. I was able to access additional research findings from reputable medical websites in America.

At a follow-up doctor's appointment I adopted a different strategy. To bolster my position, to try to gain a more positive response from the GP, I'd drawn up a list of questions. So I started by asking with pleasant politeness:

"Could an infection have moved from my bowel to my hip?"

"My dear...not since Christ was born", was his patronising response.

His doleful gaze made me wonder if he thought I was deranged.

Then he proceeded to deliver his diagnosis. It's a moment when some doctors appear to delight in using the opportunity to demonstrate their authority and superior knowledge.

"You have osteoarthritis. It's a chronic and degenerative condition caused by wear and tear. You will land up in a wheelchair and your leg muscles will waste. If you continue to take aspirin, you will run the risk of sitting on the toilet and bleeding to death."

I had originally resorted to aspirin to relieve the throbbing in my leg at night. But now the discomfort had vanished. This pronouncement left me flummoxed and speechless.

The GP ploughed on:

"Chronic means ongoing. Now what about the pain?"

But ... there was NO PAIN!

The horrific scenario that had been painted left me bewildered and confused. I found myself asking:

"But didn't you say it was tendonitis?"

"Yes, I did".

Then he confidently added as an afterthought:

"But I knew where we were going all along".

Nothing seemed to make sense, other than what the American doctor had told me.

At least I felt well and was again symptom free. The definitive diagnosis of osteoarthritis (OA) brought a certain amount of relief as it enabled me to focus my research. I could now further investigate this stealthy condition that had crept up and attacked me in the dead of night.

Possible alternative treatment

Then one morning I suddenly recalled having had a previous brush with arthritis back in 1997. As it had been more than 14 years before, and because I'd been totally symptom free, I'd completely forgotten about it. Over breakfast I mentioned this to my husband Peter and told him how I'd found a book in Fremantle's Notre Dame University library that described a doctor's effective treatment for arthritis. I had promptly bought the book and followed the advice outlined. All discomfort had disappeared in a matter of months.

When Peter heard this, his response was immediate:

"Find the book!"

After rummaging through boxes that had remained unpacked from previous moves, I eventually unearthed the book that promised a cure.

Eagerly I returned to the conservative GP where I enthusiastically produced the helpful text. After a cursory glance, and a brief flick through the pages, he pushed it back towards me. Clearly, he was unconvinced. I was taken aback, so I asked,

"Do you think this is a load of rubbish?"

"Yes" he solemnly replied, "I'm afraid I do."

This mystified me. You see, I'd not forgotten the more encouraging, positive response I'd received in 1997. My GP at that time was broadminded and approachable. He'd responded positively to the book's emphasis on a diet of largely fresh fruit and vegetables. But he also recognized that I might need the help of anti-inflammatories, so he'd given me a prescription for Celebrex. Then he'd encouraged me saying:

"Why don't you do a bit of both".

Again, I was confronted with a stark difference in medical opinions.

Chapter 4 DR CAMPBELL'S 1972 *"cure for arthritis"*

Recalling a precursor

My previous brush with arthritis in 1997 had been a short-lived experience. At that time our family had just moved back to Perth and I'd taken the opportunity to complete my post-graduate qualifications in librarianship. Fortunately, the newly established University of Notre Dame in Fremantle was expanding and looking for extra staff in their library. It turned out I was in the right place at the right time, not just to find employment, but to discover the book that was to play a crucial role in my health journey. The book written by a highly experienced osteopath was:

- Campbell, G.W., 1972: *A doctor's proven new home cure for arthritis*, Harper Collins Publishers, London, UK.

This fairly old text had been imported from the USA along with the rest of a considerable collection that Notre Dame had purchased holus-bolus.

With great enthusiasm I began work in the cavernous academic library. But initially it wasn't easy as events conspired against me and my health. As a new-comer I didn't readily fit in with the rest of the library staff who were mostly youngsters. They took a spiteful delight in harassing me. Unreasonably high standards were expected, absolutely no mistakes tolerated. To add to all the tension there were no easily accessible toilets; at least not in the vicinity of the library. You see the Catholic Church had purchased warehouses in the old port city and were in the process of converting them into university buildings. It also didn't occur to me to request a brief tea-break during my long morning shift alone at the front desk.

All of this caused my gastrointestinal tract, or gut for short, to virtually shut-down. At times there was a 10 day gap between bowel movements. As a result toxins built up in my system which resulted in inflammation, particularly in my wrists and feet. It didn't take long before I appeared arthritic.

Despite my best efforts to continue moving my hands swiftly over the computer keyboard, I simply couldn't. There was a drumming sensation in my wrists, not quite a throb, not painful, but disturbing and unpleasant.

Initially I was able to disguise that something was amiss. That was until my feet started playing up. The burning in my heels simply couldn't be ignored. At every possible opportunity I reached down and massaged them. Eventually I resorted to kicking off my shoes and rubbing my heels hard against the rough carpet. When the burning feeling spread and the entire soles of my feet started to hurt, there was no hiding the fact that I had started to hobble.

As if I hadn't already experienced enough tension and anxiety that year, yet another frightful scenario presented itself. For most arthritic conditions Campbell optimistically forecast that his approach would bring immediate relief, even a "cure". However, there was one type that he felt simply had to be addressed within the first five years of it making an appearance if joint destruction was to be prevented. This was Marie Strumpbell disease, also known as Ankylosing Spondylitis, or Spinal Arthritis.

Was I right about the hot stickiness I felt in my spine? Did this signal the start of Spinal Arthritis? Implementing Campbell's treatment became a matter of urgency, otherwise my erect posture could be permanently altered and the thought of becoming hunched over horrified me. On more than one occasion I'd seen a lonely but determined old man pushing a barrow along Stirling Highway, the busy, main thoroughfare connecting Fremantle to Perth's CBD. He'd even been featured in the local Post Newspaper. You see, he was a familiar sight amongst locals as he resembled a turtle, bent over so severely he could barely see where he was going without arching his head backwards.

All this created a sense of urgency which prompted me to take charge of my own health. I decided to follow Campbell's advice, which was surprisingly simple. All I had to do was address 3 basic bodily processes; viz.

1. Nutrition (fresh food diet with plenty of fruit & veggies)
2. Elimination (regular, ideally daily, bowel movements)
3. Circulation (lots of walking)

True to the promise on the back cover of Campbell's book, it appeared to take no time at all for my aches and pains to start disappearing. What happened one afternoon as I pushed a shopping trolley around Coles remains crystal clear in my memory. As I reached down into the deep trolley an extraordinary sensation emanated from the upper part of my spine. Again, there was that sticky feeling, but this time I felt the vertebrae coming unstuck. It was a bit like suction cups popping apart. It brought immense physical relief.

Regaining my health restored my confidence. I found myself walking with a spring in my step. It also pleased me to find I could even take in my belt a few notches. Before long I stopped taking Celebrex as there was no longer any need.

How thankful I was that the painful symptoms quietly disappeared and that I rapidly recovered. From that point on I remained vigilant; I continued to conscientiously follow Campbell's 3-step regime (see Figure 1).

All was well for many years.

Conclusion

Regrettably, it was not to last. A change of circumstances and surroundings brought with it complacency and a slide into unhealthy eating habits. During a move back to regional Australia I forgot

Campbell's guidelines and let myself go. Even my effective Herron supplements (ginseng, ginkgo biloba, cod liver oil & multivitamins) got packed away and landed up hidden at the back of a kitchen shelf.

By 2010 the lessons I'd learnt were forgotten and as discussed in chapter 2, arthritis came back in a different guise to haunt me.

Chapter 5 MULTIPLE SPECIALISTS (May 2011)

The way arthritis presented itself the second time around in 2010 was sudden. Instead of a gradual build up, the acute attacks were vicious and unbearably painful. Would I be believed, or would I again be patronizingly dismissed?

Radiologists, Rheumatologists, Gastroenterologists and Clinical Microbiologists

Without realizing it, serendipity had already stepped in to assist me. A few years earlier Peter and I had moved from suburbia to an inner-city home having become empty nesters. Our new home was perfectly located within reach of all the medical expertise I needed as Western Australia's major hospitals and research facilities were just an easy walk up the road. This was fortunate because my ability to walk freely didn't last. There was a significant alteration in my gait.

Walking like a sailor

Come April 2011 I really couldn't walk properly. No amount of leg jiggling helped. Oddly enough, it wasn't particularly painful.

In order to reassure Peter that I was "really fine", I'd gladly agreed to accompany him around the corner to mail a letter. Off we'd set and gamely I'd attempted to keep up with him. To do so meant swinging my right leg out in a most ungainly fashion. We'd barely gone 100 yards when he abruptly stopped and refused to go on, saying: "No, I'm not prepared to go with you walking like that! There's something wrong. Why are you walking like a sailor?"

From that point on things started to get a bit heated between us. Peter took the perfectly rational view that I should simply go to the doctor and get my leg fixed. Well I wasn't so sure, as I could remember shoulders being shrugged and dismissive, patronizing comments.

However, it wasn't just my sailor walk that was an issue. I now couldn't do more than one hour of ironing without a burning discomfort in my right hip forcing me to stop. I managed to get through a load of shirts by resorting to a bit of vigorous leg shaking, but it was no longer an instant solution.

Making the bed wasn't easy to do either. The burning in my hip was fierce and particularly noticeable when I had to squat down to tuck in loose blankets. I can remember gasping under my breath.

Standing for any length of time while ironing had really become a problem. My right hip wouldn't tolerate any extended weight bearing. No amount of leg shaking would stop the burning.

Before heading off to a nearby GP practice I'd decided to ask around. My gorgeous Canadian neighbour came to my rescue. I can still hear her saying,

"I go to an excellent practice in the next suburb. It's very convenient as it's on the bus route."

Referral to a radiologist

The practice my neighbour recommended was ideal as the two doctors were very experienced. I found they were also knowledgeable regarding recent advances in medicine. Possibly this was partly due to their practice being located close to WA's major medical precinct.

This time I wasn't dismissed as had happened previously. I wasn't told that "X-rays would be a waste of time and money. They won't show anything. It would unnecessarily burden an already overburdened Medicare System".

Instead, I received immediate attention. This doctor sat up and took notice. Not only was the mobility of my hip joint examined, along with the ease with which my knee could be rotated outwards, but even my reflexes were checked. A test-hammer was used to tap a tendon below my right knee cap. Questions followed regarding tingling; a feeling of pins and needles in my feet. Apparently "the integrity of my neurological functions" as well as my hip joint were being examined.

While the conscientious doctor completed his thorough examination I heard him mutter to himself,

"Mmmm ... it's the drugs ... they went public with *'it'* in the 1980s. It could be a possibility".

Then suddenly my consult was over and I was handed a referral to a radiologist to get my hip X-rayed.

As I left the surgery I wondered to myself: What was this mystery *'it'?*

That night the throbbing returned, but this time there was a new, additional symptom. I also felt slightly nauseous.

The next day Peter and I decided a lunch out would do us good. At a café overlooking the Swan River I mentioned the new symptom to him, saying,

"Whenever I swing my knee outwards, I feel sick".

I'd started to wonder whether this unwell feeling had something to do with the US doctor's diagnosis of a "cyst in my inner-hip socket".

It would take another 8 months before I found a specialist who recognized *'it'*, whatever that was, and gave me the treatment I needed.

A choice regarding treatment options

The radiologist's report was a revelation to me. As the USA doctor had predicted, my hip joint was damaged and only a thin, uneven lining of cartilage remained. A tear was noted and a large pseudocyst was spotted. Could this be the remnant of the cyst that the American doctor felt was contributing to my discomfort and interfering with my gait? Whatever the cause it now looked as though surgery was on the cards and the GP thought I'd be needing a hip replacement sooner rather than later. However, he was hesitant as I was walking normally again and not in any pain.

A referral to a rheumatologist was another option, which meant the possibility of hydrocortisone injections. To my surprise he wasn't in favour of this treatment saying,

"Hydrocortisone could increase the risk of infection by suppressing your immune system".

When infections were mentioned I instantly recalled the other piece of information from the USA doctor; viz.

"There's a major association between bowel infections and arthritis".

So I asked whether a colonoscopy might be appropriate. Without hesitation I was given a referral to see Dr Frank Brennan. It was a sliding door moment in my life as this gastroenterologist's advice would set me on a positive path to obtaining treatment not widely recognized at the time by modern, western medicine.

Referral to a gastroenterologist

Prior to my appointment with Dr Brennan I remained perplexed by the conflicting advice I'd received from doctors. Instead of being reassured, I became more apprehensive and questions flooded my mind:

- Was a gastroenterologist the type of specialist I needed to see?

- Would my "arthritis attacks" be covered by his field of medicine?
- Would he provide me with the advice I sought?

I hoped against hope that I wouldn't be turned away with the phrase: "It's not my area of expertise. I'm sorry I can't help you".

My first colonoscopy procedure in early May 2011 was a bit of an adventure, as I guess it is for most people, but my apprehension was needless. The procedure itself was over and done with while I comfortably snoozed under a duvet that had been warmed to ensure I remained cosy. But it was the preparatory procedures which I began at home, a few days ahead of time, that surprised me. Later of course I realized my gut had to be thoroughly flushed out and cleaned to ensure that anything sinister wouldn't escape being spotted.

Amongst all the hospital documentation detailing standard preparatory procedures was a questionnaire that caught my attention. It asked about arthritis, which struck me as odd. Why did the doctors in the gastroenterology department want to know whether I had arthritis?

Did these Perth doctors think there was the possibility of a link between the gut and arthritis? Maybe these gastroenterologists were collecting data with the intention of verifying such a link? Afterall, the doctor in the USA had hinted at such an association (see chapter 2).

This possible gut link was also in line with the book by Dr Campbell that I'd found in 1997 tucked away in the depths of the Notre Dame University library. He had emphasised a healthy diet to help ensure regular bowel action (see chapter 4).

These questions regarding the gut were in the forefront of my mind as I sat waiting on the hospital bed after my colonoscopy. Apparently, Dr Brennan was going to come and talk to me about the results of the procedure. It made me mildly anxious as I wondered whether this signalled a sinister discovery. However, the kind, softly spoken Irishman soon put me at ease. There was no hint of cancer on the horizon. He then went a step further. Literally on the back of an envelope he jotted down the name and address of a GP and encouraged me to,

"Go and see this doctor. He'll be able to help you. He's interested in the immune system. His practice is even close to where you live."

Conclusion

It would take another four months before I had the good fortune of obtaining an appointment with Dr Hira Singh. What was more pressing at that point in time was my need to reduce my anxiety by simply finding answers to questions regarding gastroenterology, arthritis attacks and the immune system. Up until then I'd simply been relying on the book by Dr Campbell, but then it was almost as though divine providence stepped in and my collection of texts about arthritis started to expand.

Chapter 6 DR CROOK'S 1986 THEORY

An explanatory text by William G. Crook, M.D.

The gastroenterologist's reference to the immune system left me perplexed. Was he hinting at a possible link between the gastrointestinal system, the immune system and arthritis?

It was baffling, but serendipity yet again came to my rescue. Later that week in May 2011, a dear friend popped a book in my mailbox as she passed by in the early hours on her way to work. It was almost too good to be true as the back cover of the fat tome promised a plausible explanation. Under a long list of ostensibly incurable health problems was the statement: "Psoriasis, multiple sclerosis and arthritis may be yeast connected." The book was:

- Crook, W.G., 1986: *The yeast connection.* Random House, New York, USA.

The prospect of ploughing through all 435 pages of Crook's tome was daunting. Instead, I scanned the foreword to get the gist of what he proposed. The first page zeroed in on the body's immune function. Apparently, Dr Crook had found well documented research supporting the theory that overgrowth of *Candida albicans* in the large bowel played a part in supressing the body's immune function, predisposing a patient to infections.

His book was filled with clinical evidence and case histories, which at the time I simply noted. Instead, I chose to focus on his diagrams and a flowchart which outlined a causal sequence of health issues arising from prolonged medication with broad spectrum antibiotics, cortisone and other drugs. He suggested this would contribute to the multiplication of yeasts in the gut. He illustrated how a nutritionally deficient diet with a high sugar content could start a vicious cycle, where an excessive growth of yeasts in the gut could damage the intestinal wall allowing toxins to enter the bloodstream. These toxins could result in a reaction similar to eczema.

Did Dr Crook's theory explain the two strange eczema-like patches that had appeared on my right hip and behind my right knee? Were they markers pointing to what was happening? He suggested that a flood of toxins could weaken one's immune system. Maybe something like this was affecting my right leg and was the cause of the throbbing which had disturbed my sleep?

To my mind Dr Crook provided a plausible explanation for the sensations I felt in my right leg. It was a more likely scenario than that I'd suffered some form of injury, or physical trauma. His diagrams inspired a flowchart of my own to illustrate the link between a feeble immune response that inadequately resisted infections, and disease (see Figure 2).

It then dawned on me that Dr Crook had published his ideas in 1986. Maybe this was what the GP had been thinking of when he'd muttered (see chapter 5), "It's the drugs. They went public with *'it'* in the 1980s".

Was there a theory regarding an *"Elusive it"* that doctors knew about, but that hadn't yet been proven?

William Crook wasn't the first doctor to write a book describing a "toxic condition". Dr Campbell's book which I'd obtained fourteen years earlier, contained similar advice:

- Toxic condition
- Fatigue and constipation were typical symptoms
- Treatment centred on a nutritious diet based on fresh whole-foods

Advice from a Healer and a Naturopath

Much as the doctors I'd consulted were kind and made every effort they could to help me, their cryptic clues had simply left me confused. Oddly enough it was my gardener who came to my assistance by pointing me in a useful direction.

Colin and his wife Kristina had been helping me with my gardens for many years. I'd first engaged their services when we lived in Floreat Park, a beautiful, treed suburb just inland from City Beach. They'd always made time for a friendly chat whenever they dropped by. In 2011 I discovered I'd not just been receiving the services of gardeners, but also those of a healer. For Colin, gardening was a sideline; it turned out that he mainly worked in the field of complementary health as he compassionately listened and offered advice to customers experiencing stress.

One morning as I stood poring over material I'd downloaded from the internet on GUT dysbiosis, wondering whether it was quackery or not, there was a knock on the door. It was Colin and Kristina who were passing en route to a gardening job nearby. Maybe Colin had mentioned to Kristina that I was looking for answers to puzzling health issues. Whatever the case, they arrived at an opportune time.

I also learnt that Kristina knew a bit about yeast infections. She'd battled with a shocking dose of thrush following a prolonged course of antibiotics. Now that she was fit and well, she eagerly told me to whom she'd turned to for help. It was a man she called Dr Charles, who practiced Traditional Chinese Medicine in the salubrious suburb of Dalkeith. She'd learnt from him that antibiotics could interfere with the balance of good and bad bugs in one's gut. Part of her solution had been to take probiotics.

Not entirely comfortable with the idea of trying out Traditional Chinese Medicine, I decided instead to simply seek advice from our pharmacist. As I often dropped into the large Claremont chemist for scripts, the pharmacist immediately recognised me and came over to offer assistance. Cautiously I asked him about various websites, saying:

"Ideas are outlined regarding microbial imbalance in the gut, immune dysfunction and a range of health issues. But is this information reliable?"

To my surprise he wasn't dismissive. Instead, he directed me to the naturopath's office adjacent to where a wide range of supplements were displayed.

This naturopath took me seriously. She didn't simply send me on my way with a packet full of expensive supplements. After an in-depth discussion in her office covering not just my health issues, but also my diet and lifestyle, she gave me a course of action. In addition to a pamphlet explaining dysbiosis, she provided me with a list of health practitioners. Top of her list was a homeopath whose remedies focused on natural substances. I was hesitant as I'd never before considered alternative treatments. Fortunately, she also gave me the names of two doctors whose practices were nearby. She told me that,

"These doctors knew about *'it'* and included complementary medicines in their treatments."

A mystery condition referred to as *'it'*

Yet again I'd been presented with another conundrum.

What was this *'it'*? Was it an elusive pathogen that hadn't yet been identified?

Was there more to this theory about *'it'*? When I'd asked a dermatologist, I'd learnt that *'it'* wasn't officially recognised and *'it'* wasn't taught in medical schools as *'it'* was unsubstantiated. Apparently, they were even discouraged from talking about *'it'*. No wonder she'd then condescendingly patted me on the back saying,

"I know it's frustrating when people can't help you".

I wasn't just frustrated. I was apprehensive and fearful as to what lay ahead. If there were doctors willing and able to treat *'it'*, then presumably there was a way to slow down, maybe even stop a disease that had been described earlier in the year as a "chronic and degenerative condition". The prospect of ongoing painful attacks frightened me.

Fortunately, I had someone to confide in. Someone who was interested and who understood the controversy I faced. My father-in-law, Dick, answered my telephone call. He patiently listened to my tale of confusion and then gave me the encouragement I needed.

"Mary Anne keep records; continue your investigations. I admire your determination."

Dick knew about my writing hobby. Maybe he sensed that I was embarking on a journey of discovery. A few filed notes I'd kept over the years about previous medical issues formed the basis of what was to become a detailed personal journal.

Chapter 7 BROADMINDED DOCTORS (May - Jun 2011)

Where to next? I found myself at a crossroads. Both the gastroenterologist and the naturopath had pointed me in a new direction. Intuitively I knew that if I was to uncover information regarding the mysterious *'it'*, I would have to take their advice and switch to another GP.

It wasn't a difficult choice; actually a no brainer. After all, the doctor whose practice was a short walk from our home had been recommended by two health practitioners.

In mid-May, instead of picking up the phone to make an appointment, I decided to wander up the road and within less than 5 minutes found my way to the recommended GP tucked away in an old house in a quiet corner of Nedlands.

Dr Hira Singh was special. I felt that from the moment I saw him step out of his consulting room. He had a calm, gentle aura, coupled with assurance and there was the added touch of mystique because he wore a turban. He was a Sikh who practiced Integrative Medicine.

Unfortunately, at that moment my attempts to find the help I needed were again stalled. When I approached the friendly receptionist to make an appointment I was told,

"I'm sorry Dr Singh is fully booked for the next 4 months, but I can get you an appointment with his partner."

Dr Singh's young colleague cheerily greeted me and asked why I'd come to see him. I'm sure he wasn't expecting the torrent of information that hit him. The medical establishment's apparent inability to recognise my condition had made me resort to looking for information and help on the internet. Was it any wonder that by the time I met this young doctor I was in overdrive?

My new-found knowledge meant I'd gone armed to the doctor's surgery with a clear outline of my symptoms and why I felt (in both senses of the word) I had *Septic Arthritis.* I also now had my first CT Scan and report describing "Advanced, degenerative arthrosis of the right hip."

The young doctor probably felt beleaguered and had to beg me to stop talking so he could carefully read the radiologist's report. He also looked at my notes. Then he asked whether I could walk and half-laughed, saying "but of course you can, you just walked in here."

Remember by that stage I'd received a course of macrodantin and was "walking freely". So for the life of me I couldn't see why he initially suggested I needed to be managed by an orthopaedic surgeon and had handed me a referral.

But imagine my relief when he hesitated and after a few moments of quiet thought, the young GP suddenly looked up at me and said:

"What about seeing a microbiologist? Dr Clay Golledge at the Hollywood Specialist Centre will know. He's world renowned and has more than 20 years' experience."

Armed with a referral to see an infectious disease specialist, I headed for home. But when I got through to the specialist's receptionist I was told he was heavily booked; they'd call me back if a cancellation became available. Obtaining an appointment wasn't going to be straightforward.

Another full-blown, excruciating attack

A week later I experienced another unbelievably excruciating attack. It made the previous one, where I'd swung my leg in all directions, pale into insignificance. Again I was woken in the middle of the night. This time there was a sharp severe pain at the top of my right foot, just below my ankle. It made me gasp it was so intense. In an instant I was scrunched in a foetal position and I found myself digging my thumbs into the burning spot on my foot. That was the only way to make the extreme pain bearable. If only I could've made it stop.

Besides the sharp pain in my foot, my knee ached too. No finger pressure or massage would ease the discomfort there. Again, the best I could do was to press my knee into the mattress in an effort to ease the throbbing.

There was no more sleep to be had that night. At daybreak the pain had vanished, but this time the memory of it caused tears to roll down my cheeks. However, it was a normal working day for Peter. The kettle went on and a quick breakfast was downed, before he headed out the door. As I didn't want to distress him, I didn't breathe a word about what had transpired in the night.

Fortunately, though, there was someone to confide in. Susan, my sister, happened to be staying with us for a few days. She found my story of such extreme pain quite strange. Was I exaggerating? Had I just dreamt it, or was it all a figment of my imagination? Surely this couldn't be, as I was comfortably standing there in the kitchen pain free. Aghast, she responded with incredulous amazement, "but Mary Anne, maybe your blankets are too heavy?"

My sister's response dented my self-confidence. Was I nuts to have imagined such excruciating pain? Could it simply be put down to blankets that were too heavy? No, this could not be. Evidently what I'd experienced was beyond my sister's comprehension.

It must be hard to imagine such pain unless one's actually experienced it. There again, I too cannot really recall the pain, just my response to it.

Of course, I wondered whether this was the pain I'd been asked about earlier in the year? The conservative GP had warned me that my OA condition was chronic, which meant ongoing. Was this what lay ahead; frightful, excruciating nightly attacks? Suddenly I felt a desperate need to find more help, other than the Nurofen that had been recommended.

Back I went to see the young doctor. This time I had the comfort of my sister's company, but it was all the comfort to be had. When doctors don't really know, it's a case of shrugging shoulders, or shaking heads.

"Maybe it was referred pain?" was the best explanation he could offer.

All of this just heightened my tension as I'd yet to secure an appointment with Dr Clay Golledge. A phone call was then made by the GP and to my great relief I was given a time to see the clinical microbiologist the following week.

An appointment with a microbiologist (infectious disease specialist)

I desperately hoped my frightening experience wouldn't be beyond the knowledge and understanding of Dr Golledge. With the hope of gaining some clarification I drew up a list of the questions that were at the forefront of my mind:

- What had caused the extremely intense pain?
- Why was it short-lived/acute?
- Why did those acute attacks occur in the middle of the night?
- Would these attacks be "ongoing" as I'd been told?
- Would it affect other joints?
- Could the underlying cause be identified and treated?
- Could this *arthritis* be stopped?

A quick walk the following week took me to the consulting rooms of a great many doctors located in the Hollywood Specialist centre. There I spotted Dr Golledge's name listed on the second floor and in no time at all I found myself in a comfortable waiting room.

The specialist soon appeared and ushered me into his surgery. His approach from the outset brought a sense of relief. There were no patronising put-downs. Instead he listened to my story and gave me a sense that he understood. He also checked the eczema-like patches on my right hip and behind my right knee. However, when it came to my questions there were no clear answers. Like the GP he talked about surgical interventions.

As I was still "walking freely" and without pain I simply couldn't entertain the prospect of major surgery. I think Dr Golledge understood; he didn't pressure me. Instead, he advised against excessive use of Nurofen (apparently it damages the liver) and gave me a prescription for Voriconazole; a strong antifungal.

Chapter 8 GUT HEALTH RESTORED (Jun – Jul 2011)

At the beginning of June 2011 a cloud of uncertainty hung over me. Should I immediately take the strong antifungal I'd been prescribed or should I first try the Claremont naturopath's suggestion and seek out a natural homeopathic option?

I was in a quandary and it was my sister who helped me make a decision. She'd returned to her home in Melbourne where she hadn't simply let matters rest. Aware of my anxiety and suffering, she'd called a close friend to get some advice. Her friend Andrea had completed a five year course in Chinese Medicine. This was my good fortune, as I'd learnt from another doctor that apparently Chinese Medicine is more advanced than Western Medicine when it comes to treating chronic diseases. Andrea immediately suggested acupuncture.

A Western Medical Practice that included Chinese Medicine

As I'd never heard of acupuncture - no doctor had ever suggested it to me - I wondered where I should seek such treatment. A dear friend provided me with the answer by urging me to contact her GP, whom she highly recommended. Apparently, his practice covered both Modern Medicine and Traditional Chinese Medicine. He also understood the importance of Gut Health as he was a functional medicine doctor.

However, my friend warned me the tests and treatments would be costly as most of it would not be covered by Medicare. Yet in spite of the cost, her doctor's services were in high demand. I couldn't readily make an appointment. Instead, I had to ask to be put on a waiting list in the hope of a cancellation.

As time was of the essence, I decided to unearth the empty Herron bottles from 1997 that had once contained helpful supplements. There was no doubt in my mind that during those difficult months at the library in Freo, my collection of capsules taken at brekky had been beneficial.

When I arrived at Woolies the following day I was disappointed to find the rows of Herron supplements had been replaced with products by Nature's Way. I suspected that the tried and trusted Australian brand had been bought out, but this really wasn't a problem as I was able to select 5 bottles that promised to boost my general health:

1. Cod Liver Oil
2. Multivitamins
3. Ginkgo Biloba
4. Ginseng
5. Odourless Garlic

I'd never taken capsules of garlic before but my trusty father-in-law, Dick had recommended it, so I thought I'd give it a try.

Dysbiosis

Both Dr Giraud Campbell and Dr William Crook had described a toxic condition as a possible source of my arthritic attacks. Even though some doctors had dismissed this theory, I remained hopeful that my friend's GP might be more receptive to the idea. Before my first appointment I decided to go armed with the 2 texts that had given me hope.

- Campbell, G.W., 1972: *A doctor's proven new home cure for arthritis*, Harper Collins Publishers, London, UK.
- Crook, W.G., 1986: *The yeast connection.* Random House, New York, USA.

So my sense of relief was palpable when this doctor acknowledged that the cause of my frightful attacks was likely to be a toxic condition linked to dysbiosis. Not only had I found a GP who acknowledged that some of the content in Campbell and Crook's books was worthwhile, he'd also validated that the information I'd found on the internet about dysbiosis wasn't quackery. In fact, a severe toxic imbalance of bacteria in the gut could cause serious gastro-intestinal infections. What he then told me took my breath away. With cases of deadly colitis, doctors used a treatment called faecal microbiota transplantation. This procedure has been known for more than 50 years and was previously called faecal bacteriotherapy. Today it's informally called a stool transplant.

Fortunately, my case wasn't deadly. However, the first test this friendly, broadminded GP requested required a stool sample. It was at the top of quite a list that also included:

- Urine test
- Saliva test
- Blood test (Thyroid function)
- Adrenocortex Stress Test (Adrenal Gland function)
- Hair tissue mineral analysis
- MRI scan of my right leg

At this point he ran out of time, but to ensure I left his surgery with all necessary information he handed me a few information sheets. They covered,

1. Vitamin D
2. Detoxification and Dysbiosis

To my delight I discovered I was already on the right track, as the Cod Liver Oil encouraged by Campbell was mentioned as a good dietary source of Vitamin D. It even stated research findings which showed that,

"Low vitamin D increases one's risk of *rheumatoid arthritis*."

This doctor was of the opinion that the role vitamin D played was critically important. Straight away he started me on a large daily dose, by providing me with 2 bottles of Vitamin D3 sourced from a New Zealand company called "Integrative Medicine Ltd".

The rest of the information about dysbiosis I could finish reading at home before returning in 2 weeks' time. By then all the test results would be in and treatment would commence to restore my gut health.

Detoxification Program

The treatment plan I was to follow over the next two months had similarities with the stool transplant procedure. It would be a 2-part program that aimed at achieving 5 outcomes:

1. Removal of hostile organisms (harmful bacteria, fungi and parasites)
2. Replacement with beneficial probiotics
3. Restoration of gut health and gut lining repair
4. Improvement of waste removal
5. Enhancement of the Immune System

Point 4 was the same as a key criterion of Campbell's; viz. "Elimination!"

Gut Health Treatment

Towards the end of June 2011 I started a detoxification program. It was quite complex, involving an assortment of pills, powders and potions. But again this doctor was organised and provided me with another information sheet outlining exactly what to take and at what time of the day. In addition there were dietary guidelines; e.g. a high fibre diet, plenty of fruit and vegetables, less sugar, yeast, bread and processed foods.

This time I recognised advice not just similar to Dr Campbell's, but also to Dr Crook's. Even Nystatin, a drug trumpeted in his book "The Yeast Connection", was listed.

As the program progressed I noticed beneficial changes. My bowel movements had become regular and I sensed that my gut was healing. What was also clearly noticeable was that the unpleasant, prickling and niggling sensations in my right leg steadily dissipated. What remained though was the impact the attack had had on my muscles. My right leg had become significantly weaker than my left. I could no longer use it to step onto the kitchen stool I used to reach top shelves. Undeterred I started my own exercise routine, beginning with simple leg raises.

By the time of my final appointment at the detoxification clinic in early August, I'd remarkably improved. The GP's advice and therapy in the treatment of my arthritis with essentially natural methods had been very effective.

Eager to further clarify what I'd experienced, I asked if there was an explanation for the prickling sensations that had vanished. This is what I was told:

"When muscles become inflamed pressure on nerves can cause tingling; an unpleasant condition called paraesthesia. Sometimes nerves can even become pinched which can be agonising."

This doctor's explanations and treatment had helped me to relax as I felt another painful attack was no longer imminent. However, I still wondered why he'd recommended I delay taking Dr Golledge's antifungal until his treatment had been completed. Apparently:

"Voriconazole deals with harmful microorganisms in one's bloodstream and tissues, whereas the detoxification treatment targeted the GUT."

Another major question still remained. Was surgery needed? The GP's reply delighted me:

"If you continue to improve you don't have to see an orthopaedic surgeon."

This encouraging news prompted me to ask whether his treatment meant I was cured. Unfortunately, yet another riddle was presented.

"Look I've had *'it'*. We can stabilise *'it'*, but we can't repair."

Again I was left completely baffled. The search for *'it'*; the challenge to figure out what *'it'* was continued.

Eventually I would land up working out my own theoretical explanation, as it appeared no doctor was prepared to come up with a definitive answer. Once I'd formulated my own understanding I would, 10 years on, obtain another MRI to establish whether the functional medicine doctor was correct. Had my arthritic condition indeed been stabilised?

Chapter 9 PHYSIOTHERAPY REHABILITATION (Aug 2011)

Once the detoxification treatment was completed, I felt confident that my gut health had been restored. It was greatly reassuring as my gut function had dramatically improved; comfortable daily bowel movements occurred as a matter of course. It was smooth sailing.

With the restoration of gut health came the reassurance that it was likely my gut lining had been strengthened because toxic organisms and severe constipation were no longer damaging my bowel wall. With the barrier function of my intestines restored I could confidently assume toxins were no longer seeping into my bloodstream and overwhelming my immune system. I felt confident that those excruciating "arthritis attacks" had been stopped.

I was now determined not to forget the lessons I'd relearnt and that the dietary guidelines I'd been given would remain front of mind for the rest of my life. This would help to ensure that the integrity of my bowel was maintained.

Even though a lot of my questions had been answered by the GP who practiced functional medicine, I still didn't have a clear grasp of what *'it'* was. But what was important was his encouragement, which restored my confidence. I felt that I was no longer groping in the dark.

After-effects of major attack

The detoxification treatment of the imbalance of microflora in my gut had been remarkably effective. My right leg remained pain free;

throbbing had ceased; even unpleasant, prickly niggles that I'd sensed from hip to toe had vanished.

However, I'd noticed a significant change in my agility, even though I continued to walk freely. It was no longer easy for me to cut my toenails. Touching my toes had become difficult and, as already mentioned, my right leg had become significantly weaker than my left. I couldn't lift it up to step onto the kitchen stool I used to reach top shelves. It was distressing to find that practically overnight I'd become saddled with a gammy, 'stick-like' right leg.

Enfeebled by acute "arthritic attacks"

These after-effects of the second attack frightened me. The pain had passed, but I was left disabled. My right leg was so weak I had to use both hands to lift it up onto a footrest when relaxing in front of the TV. Household chores that I'd done without thinking, now became mammoth tasks. My left leg had to take the load because when I bent over the right stick-leg had to be swung stiffly backwards. Spontaneous bending over to remove stray weeds that popped up between the pavers had become a habit of the past. Our once tidy courtyards now took on an air of neglect as weeds flourished.

The attacks had ended. The functional medicine doctor correctly predicted that my condition would be "stabilised", but I was left puzzled by the fact that they "couldn't repair".

What I then learnt from a friend left me puzzled and disturbed. In her splendid, modern inner-city home there were three flights of stairs. Neither bedroom, nor bathroom were located on the ground floor. She told me that the previous owners of her new home had to sell when: "She got arthritis."

Our main bedroom and bathroom also had to be reached by going up a flight of stairs. The prospect of selling our home, which we loved, confronted me. Once stricken, would I become permanently debilitated? Maybe the awful prognosis I'd been given in April 2011 was correct after all?

Nevertheless, I remained stubbornly determined. I wasn't going to let that prognosis become a reality if I could help it. Again, it was my sister who lent a helping hand when a birthday book from her appeared in my letterbox. Coincidentally it described the case of a stroke victim who was pig-headed and obstinately refused to accept that he would remain lame. He defied the prognosis he was given. As a result, a startling medical concept was developed called "brain plasticity".

- Doidge, N., 2015: *The brain's way of healing,* Viking Penguin, New York, USA.

Dr Norman Doidge's book recounted medical success stories of patients who'd remarkably recovered. It startled me to learn that for 400 years the mainstream medical view of the brain was that it could not change. This view was countered in 1948 when a Polish neuroscientist coined the term "neuroplasticity". What also intrigued me was that Dr Doidge, in a matter-of-fact manner, referred in his preface to a condition called "intestinal permeability". To my mind this scotched the notion that infections couldn't move from the bowel to the hip. Further on in his book he expanded on the well known "placebo effect" and a lesser known "nocebo response". Basically, a patient's symptoms could worsen if a doctor's prognosis lowered their expectations. False despair could be inadvertently harmful.

My simple home exercise program

The mantra "use it or lose it" now remained front of mind. Undeterred I started my own exercise routine, beginning with simple knee raises. Soon I was rewarded with the satisfaction of being able to place my right heel on my left knee with ease, while balancing on one leg. This I first did while standing at the kitchen counter, which wasn't ideal. So my home exercises increased to a program consisting of 4 sets, each in a different location in our home.

1. Lower staircase step: The position at the base of our staircase was ideal as the firm stainless-steel handrails on either side provided stability and support. Here I did step-ups & step downs, alternating between my strong left leg and the weak right one.
2. Foot stool: The foot stool exercise, consisting of leg raises without using my hands, was simply carried out before relaxing in front of the TV at the end of the day. I persisted until once again I could effortlessly swing my foot up onto the footrest.
3. Knee-high shower wall: Stepping over the low wall into our shower recess was a challenge. At first I had to turn sideways to get into our shower/bath. Eventually I stepped over and in without thinking.
4. Lying down on my bed: The bed exercise was easy and pleasantly relaxing. All I had to do was lie on my back, bend my knees and envisage that a huge porridge pot was positioned between my feet. "Pot-stirring" would then commence; first with the left leg and then with the right. I pictured my lower leg as a large wooden spoon with my heel as the scoop.

This simple exercise program soon rewarded me with the satisfaction of slowly but surely attaining each of my goals. The possibility of having to move house began to recede. Even my ability to climb upstairs with swift, sprightly ease returned, as did the ease with which I again raised my right leg high to step over our knee-high shower wall. It was particularly gratifying to eventually be able to balance on either my left or my right leg. Who would've thought I'd master balancing stock still on my once feeble right leg to the count of ten?

Practical, self-help texts

Memories of walking like a sailor were fading. With the strength in my right leg restored, I was again able to accompany Peter on our 10 minute walk to the Nedlands Library, which is part of the Western Suburbs Library Network and provides a wonderful, free service to the local community.

On entering the two-storey building, Peter and I automatically gravitated towards the well-stocked, 'just in' shelves close to the entry. Even though I felt well on the way to recovery, my curiosity remained as there were questions that I still hoped to find answers to. So my attention was quickly drawn to two new books with strikingly similar covers. These recent publications came from the UK and were published by "How to books Ltd." in Oxford. They were both self-help guides for arthritis patients containing lots of information about the condition, as well as practical advice on how to move on with one's life:

- Jenkins, J., 2011: *Rheumatoid arthritis; a self-help guide to getting on with your life*, How To Books Ltd, Oxford, UK
- Jenner, C., 2011: *Arthritis; a practical guide to getting on with your life*, How To Books Ltd, Oxford, UK.

Jasmine Jenkins's book provided a lot of personal advice as she'd lived with rheumatoid arthritis for more than 30 years. What I found helpful was the information she included that covered additional, supportive therapies she'd found beneficial; therapies her GP didn't offer.

Dr Chris Jenner's credentials were impressive, as he was an authority in the field of arthritis with a practice in Harley Street, London. As I began reading the opening chapter of his book I felt as though he'd stood in my shoes. He described exactly the issues I'd hit up against, such as the grim prognosis I'd been given early on in the year. He predicted my anxiety caused by the fear of what might lie ahead of me. He ended the chapter by strongly recommending that patients take control of their health. Instead of restricting themselves to the advice and help of a single health practitioner, they should consider additional supportive techniques and therapies.

What Dr Jenner proposed was a holistic, multidisciplinary approach. His advice and encouragement was like manna from heaven, as further on in his book he stated:

"in some cases it's possible to drive arthritis into complete remission."

By that stage I'd already received treatment from the functional medicine doctor, whose clinic encompassed some ancient, Chinese healing therapies. So I turned my attention to other supportive treatments. Realising how beneficial my simple home exercises had been, I thought that it was time for me to become a bit more ambitious. Maybe I should expand my home exercise program?

From Jenkins's book I learnt that, in addition to strengthening muscles, exercise could also improve flexibility and range-of-motion, as well as increase blood circulation. However, her advice came together with a word of caution. She recommended that patients should obtain guidance from a professional, such as a physiotherapist, who would be able to determine an appropriate exercise program. One that would be co-ordinated and safe.

Physiotherapy rehabilitation

Living within a medical precinct again proved advantageous. Just a five-minute walk up the road from my home was a practice that advertised "Physio based rehabilitation". So, towards the end of August, I wandered up the street and entered such a practice for the 1st time. As I arrived, a pilates class was just ending and I had to make way for a bevy of lithe young women who were emerging; gaily chattering amongst each other. As a late middle-aged woman approaching 60 I felt a bit out of place, and wondered whether this physio practice would be suitable for me.

However, my fears were unfounded. The lovely young physio immediately suggested a one hour consult so she could make an assessment of my issues and determine how to address them. She assured me that, with the right exercises, I'd restore and maintain normal gait and posture.

A personalised exercise plan

By the end of the session the physiotherapist had equipped me with a personalised exercise plan tailored to my needs. I was provided with exercise sheets covering all sorts of moves. Some were not unlike my own home program. However, I was cautioned to be careful when using exercises that move the leg away from the body. I should avoid extreme rotation of the hips. That signalled the end of my 'pot stirring' exercise. Instead, I learnt that any sensation of tightness in my hip should be teased out gently and very gradually. The 'femur circles' she recommended were smaller. Instead of a huge porridge pot, I should envisage drawing a dinner plate in the air.

There was no need for me to attend regular sessions after that as I'd completed the comprehensive set of exercises and been equipped with guidelines. The easy-to-follow movements could become part of an extended home programme. I was relieved to know there'd be no need for me to match the flexible, lithe young ladies.

At home I began the discipline of a more extensive exercise program, confident that all agility would be restored. But I hit up against a problem. The very last exercise listed was a 'standing roll down'. This was still not possible. Those weeds in the garden were to remain for the time being. Spontaneously swooping down to pluck weeds from between pavers was still out of the question. The ability to touch my toes continued to elude me.

Chapter 10 TREATMENT FOR RESIDUAL DISCOMFORT (Sept 2011)

In September 2011 I continued to be confronted with the problem of stiffness in my right hip joint and my inability to cut my toenails. Thankfully fate intervened when a letter appeared in my mailbox which came from the clinic recommended to me by the gastroenterologist.

In the same way as Dr Jenner's advice had resonated with me, so did Dr Hira Singh's. In his letter he stressed "whole person care" and emphasised "empowering the patient through the use of an educational approach". Together with the letter was a flyer covering the wide range of physiotherapy services also offered at the clinic. Dry-needling was listed on the flyer as a "highly effective technique" used to ease arthritic symptoms.

In Dr Jenner's chapter on "non-pharmaceutical treatments" he'd stressed that a holistic approach to the treatment of arthritis was proving to be more effective than standard, more limited treatment. However, he emphasised that patients must ensure that these additional healthcare providers were properly trained and qualified. He went on to discuss the benefits of acupuncture. Apparently recent scientific research had produced very positive results, as it had been found that this technique significantly improved joint function.

Dr Singh's letter indicated that, like the functional medicine doctor, his practice also offered a wide range of additional supportive techniques, therapies and supplements. As his clinic was less than a 5 minute walk away from my home it was very conveniently located. This prompted me to recontact his surgery.

Vitamin D3 and Cod Liver Oil

The functional medicine doctor had supplied me with a large bottle of high dose vitamin D3 capsules and I still had some left over once his treatment was completed. He'd recommended I finish using them and encouraged me to continue taking vitamin D3 for the rest of my life, particularly as I was close to 60 years of age. So when the bottle was almost empty, instead of heading off to the supermarket, I walked down Broadway to a local health store. This turned out to be a wise move.

The health store was well stocked and there was plenty of choice. More importantly the young man in the store was exceedingly helpful. I learnt that not all supplements were equally reliable, because complementary products weren't subjected to the same regulations as pharmaceutical medicines. He went on to recommend liquid Cod Liver Oil sourced from New Zealand, rather than the supermarket capsules I'd purchased earlier in the year.

While completing my purchase we chatted a bit about my health issues and where I'd found help. I mentioned how difficult it had been to obtain an appointment with Dr Singh. According to the young man, this was because he'd stopped taking new patients. When I told him about the letter I'd received, his response left me quite certain as to the next step I would take. He urged me to try making another appointment saying, "He's an excellent doctor. You are very lucky!"

All the while, I continued to inform myself so I could take more control of my own health. The next text I found in the local library proved to be an absolute mine of useful information:

- Weatherby, C. and Gordin, L., 1999: *The Arthritis Bible,* Healing Arts Press, Rochester, USA.

This book expanded my understanding of holistic physicians and additional treatment options. Apparently these doctors were knowledgeable about supportive therapies, but their training grounded them in medical science. I discovered that Dr Hira Singh was such a physician; a medical doctor who used a holistic approach and was also a skilled acupuncturist. He was a GP trained and experienced in Integrative Medicine.

Help from a qualified and experienced physiotherapist and acupuncturist

Without any further delay, I gave Dr Singh's surgery a call. This time I was in luck as I was immediately able to make two appointments: a physiotherapy appointment the following week and one with the doctor towards the end of September.

Aware that GPs can be curtailed by time constraints, I understood why the functional medicine doctor had been super-efficient. However, my experience with the previous physiotherapist had been different. There'd been more time to address my queries, no matter how trivial. With this in mind, I went well prepared for my next physio appointment. I drew up a list of questions, included a newspaper article on the benefits of cod liver oil and then tucked my X-rays from the scan in April under my arm. In addition I included my journal of "Pain Records". In Jenkins's book she'd mentioned that such record-keeping could well be useful.

Early on the Monday morning I arrived in good time to find the old-fashioned surgery bustling with activity. Fortunately, one seat remained vacant. While I waited, I absorbed the feel of the practice and found it strangely soothing. Instead of blank walls there were paintings, the one I particularly loved being of Freshwater Bay, part of a sweeping bend in the Swan River. Behind the receptionist's wooden counter, which had a warm patina reflecting decades of use, was a backdrop of Jarrah shelving filled to bursting point with patients' records collected over more than 40 years.

Before long a charming young person appeared. She extended her hand and warmly introduced herself. This was the physiotherapist who was an expert at dry-needling. Most of the room where the physiotherapist practiced was occupied by a massage table and to the side were shelves stacked with fresh, white towels. But there was space against the wall for a desk and a couple of comfortable chairs. Seated there alongside her I learnt a lot more about my condition and the possible source of those horrific attacks. She wasn't reluctant to elaborate and openly shared her knowledge based on observational clinical evidence.

I began by showing her the article from *The Australian* newspaper titled,

"The Pulse. The latest medical research from around the world."

She was interested to learn that recent arthritis research findings from Britain showed a reduction in the destruction of joint cartilage amongst patients who took cod liver oil, and promptly asked to photocopy it!

We moved on to my X-rays which she pinned to a light-backed board for ease of viewing. As far as possible I wanted to understand what I felt, so it pleased me that she was able to quickly identify the key features described in the radiologist's report; viz. damaged hip cartilage (only a thin lining remained) and a large pseudo-cyst. Turning to me she gave an explanation which made perfect sense:

"You've had an infection and your joint has been damaged".

Explanations provided by doctors earlier in the year had been "wear and tear", or "inflammation". Yet information on page one of *The Arthritis Bible* stated that periodic inflammations weren't a feature of OA, which was a slow, degenerative disease. No, the physiotherapist's explanation sounded a lot more plausible.

I then referred to my Pain Records, which really had become more of a record of sensations in my right leg, rather than excruciating attacks. However, back in April I'd told a white lie which I decided to share with this helpful physio. When the GP had asked me whether I was experiencing tingling in my leg, or a feeling of pins and needles in my feet, I'd simply shaken my head in denial. Now that the unpleasant condition called paraesthesia had receded thanks to the functional medicine doctor, I no longer minded sharing this information. I even shared a bothersome secret, that three of the toes on my right foot were numb.

Immediately I was asked to remove my socks and shoes so she could have a closer look. She also asked me to press my toes down onto her fingers, which revealed a curiosity. The two toes next to my big toe were quite floppy. They had no rigidity at all.

My floppy toes didn't alarm this self-assured physio who promptly formed a tight roll with a small towel which she tucked under my toes. She then told me to clench my toes around the roll as tightly as possible, reassuring me that I would regain the lost firmness if I kept up the exercise. Besides that I shouldn't worry about it.

Of course, I was left wondering whether some neurological function or other had been compromised. Possibly, like Dr Doidge, this physio was aware of the phenomenon known as neuroplasticity and that rehabilitation should not be discounted. I didn't expect miracles. I'd be happy with a partial restoration of the strength of my toes and from then on I made every effort to improve my toes' strength. Those exercises became part and parcel of my plan to assist my body's capacity to self-repair where possible.

My Pain Records were then again referred to by the physiotherapist. On the previous Saturday Peter and I had strolled down to Matilda Bay. With my leg steadily strengthening, we'd been able to resume this lovely, 10 minute walk through the gardens on the university campus. However, the notes in my journal indicated I'd encountered some bothersome issues:

- 3rd September 2011 – Walk irritated right leg nerve; quite painful; required rest
- Limping that night at JD's birthday dinner

After a quick assessment of my gait and joint flexibility, she gave me an encouraging response.

"I may be able to fix this problem."

A follow up appointment for 'nerve treatment' was made; the 2nd of 5 appointments that the Medicare scheme allotted for joint rehabilitation. Three days later when I returned, that next appointment marked a turning point.

While relaxed on the massage table I had my first experience of Dry-Needling. It took me by surprise as I didn't anticipate that this therapy would cause me to revisit the major attack I'd endured in May. I again experienced a sharp, fierce pain at my ankle, but thank goodness this time it was only fleeting! That very uncomfortable pinched nerve down my leg still led to a burning point above my foot. Thankfully an initial, brief shock was quickly ameliorated with a follow-up massage which was gentle and comforting.

Once the treatment was over, this amazing physiotherapist asked me to roll onto my back, sit up and touch my toes. Well, I thought that it might be a tall ask, but without further ado I did exactly that. In an instant suppleness and flexibility had been restored. It was extraordinary!

Even though the acupuncture and dry-needling mechanisms aren't fully understood and don't work for everyone, the reduction in my pain and stiffness was undeniable. It appeared to have had a neurological effect, perhaps by removing muscle tension, releasing nerve pressure and increasing blood flow. Whatever the case, flexibility was restored and I've remained supple and agile ever since.

My October entry in my pain journal recorded:

- No discomfort when cutting toenails
- Sprightly walk with K!
- R. leg no longer stiff!

Thermal Ultrasound Therapy

Having eased the stiffness in my right hip and stopped the sharp twinge at my ankle, the physiotherapist then turned her attention to my knee; the one that had throbbed at night and disturbed my sleep in April/May. Apparently there was no further need for 'nerve treatment', but my knee did require a different type of therapy to assist in its full recovery, as it was likely that tissues in and around the joint had been damaged.

At my third appointment I received Thermal Ultrasound Therapy which to my delight, I found warm and soothing. First of all a gel was smoothed over my knee. Then a hand-held device was gently moved in a constant circular motion over the area that had throbbed. While doing so the physiotherapist explained that the mild pulses I felt were sound waves penetrating the tissues, increasing metabolism and promoting healing.

Once the therapy was completed, my knee was firmly strapped and remained that way until I returned for a follow-up massage. A final review of strength and joint flexibility followed and it was as though a little miracle had occurred. I was once again agile and supple. With the tension around my right hip joint gone, my ability to carry out my own pedicure had been restored, and nothing was wrong with my gait. This marked the start of more frequent and longer walks with Peter along the banks of the Swan.

Answers to remaining questions

All of the physio's therapies had been extraordinarily beneficial and left me wanting to share my experience with other arthritis sufferers. So before my final appointment I made a note of a few more questions. If possible I hoped to gain a better understanding of the symptoms I'd experienced and the treatment I'd received.

- *I began by asking why back in April the GP had finished his examination of my right leg by using a test-hammer to check my reflexes.*

The reply was simple: "MS would be my guess."

Thankfully she immediately reassured me that my "attack" was part of the infection and not actual MS; i.e. my tingling was caused by inflamed muscles putting pressure on nerves.

She then reminded me to keep up with my toe exercises and I like to think that ten years on, the wonderful physiotherapist would be pleased I took heed and followed her advice. My right toes are by and large firm, although not quite the same as those on my left. Any sensations of tingling are long forgotten.

- *I then asked how the acupuncture/dry-needling "nerve treatment" had brought about such instant and remarkable relief.*

Even though acupuncture isn't fully understood, I was given a plausible explanation. Apparently when my hip's range of movement (ROM) was initially assessed, restriction was found due to muscle tightness. Some muscles were in spasm and intense dry-needling was needed for them to relax. Basically the neuro-muscular therapy had relayed messages to the nervous system, resulting in reduced muscle tension. This relieved nerve compression and resulted in the miraculous improvement.

- *Why then had I not been referred to a physiotherapist earlier in the year?*

Apparently Dr Singh was a GP who, in addition to his knowledge of western medicine, had received a broader training in Integrative Medicine, which included non-pharmaceutical therapies. So he was accustomed to the option of referring arthritis patients for physiotherapy.

- *I'd already received largely non-pharmaceutical therapy from a functional medicine doctor. Was this treatment sufficient?*

Should I disregard Dr Golledge's prescription for Voriconazole?

"This is something you need to talk through with Dr Singh. But what I can provide you with is a report covering the results of my treatment."

In no time at all a report was typed up and signed. I would land up bringing it to Dr Golledge's attention before the year was out.

Once the physio's therapies had been completed, it was immensely satisfying for me to make three additional notes in my Pain Record:

- Strength in right leg restored
- Easy, free movement
- Striding out with confidence

To have received such beneficial treatment was a privilege. Yet it left me feeling concerned that such help wasn't more widely known about. It was only thanks to luck that I lived so close to where the help I sought was to be found. In my opinion overcoming arthritic discomfort shouldn't be left to chance and that such beneficial healthcare shouldn't be a matter of luck.

Chapter 11 INTEGRATIVE MEDICINE (Oct 2011)

On my return to the small "Whole Health Clinic" at the end of Hardy Road, I found a little miracle had been performed. Prior to my first appointment with Dr Hira Singh at the end of September 2011, I felt hugely satisfied and confident in the knowledge that my right leg had been largely restored to how it was before the onslaught of arthritis attacks; i.e. nerve pressure released, tissues repaired and muscles strengthened. Overall balance and posture had been corrected. Limping and "sailor-walking" had become a thing of the past. Surely surgery would no longer be on the cards?

A GP trained in Integrative Medicine

Conflicting advice from doctors since the start of 2011 had heightened stress levels; not just mine, but Peter's too. We both felt major surgery wasn't necessary at that stage. Instead Dr Jenner had emphasised in his book that a holistic approach was needed in order to get to the bottom of my issues, which of course included stress levels. It turned out that Jenner, the Harley Street doctor, was absolutely right.

Upon entering Dr Singh's office I instantly felt soothed by his calm presence. This is what my sister had described as his "special aura". In May we'd been able to observe the gentle Sikh as he calmly moved from receptionist, to patient, to his office where a solid jarrah door was closed ensuring total privacy. Instinctively I knew that this time there would be no need for me to assert myself in order to be given the attention I sought.

Instead of simply being told to take ibuprofen and then being handed a referral to see an orthopaedic surgeon, Dr Singh adopted a totally different approach. Besides questions regarding any residual discomfort, my disturbed sleep was also noted. However, painkillers and sleeping tablets weren't prescribed. To the contrary, these drugs were firmly discouraged. Not only could prolonged use be harmful, but there was also the serious danger of addiction. From this wise doctor I learnt about safer, more natural options.

Sitting there with Dr Singh I was to learn what an integrative approach meant. Instead of the focus being on symptoms, attention was turned to what else might be troubling me. Why was I disturbed? Why was I not sleeping well?

The philosophy behind Integrative Medicine (IM) was then clearly explained. I learnt that IM doctors not only treat troubling symptoms but are also interested in preventing further arthritic disease. Furthermore, the patient is viewed as a whole person, which means aspects such as what is on one's mind and one's emotional state are also taken into account. Dr Singh took a sheet of paper and calmly and clearly outlined how stress could impact on overall health. For me this holistic concept was new, so I was grateful to be given his annotated diagram. It made me realise that many factors were involved.

The start of Comprehensive Preventative Treatment

Having provided me with an understanding that several variables were at play, it was down to business. As there were many factors which needed to be addressed, I came to understand that a single magic bullet, a drug that was a cure-all didn't exist. To increase my chances of preventing further painful attacks I would need Dr Singh's guidance.

To begin with, the medications, vitamins, minerals and herbs I took were listed. I mentioned the five products I'd recently purchased from the health store. Dr Singh readily approved of the vitamins I took, but he wasn't totally comfortable about Ginkgo Biloba, a herb he was familiar with. Apparently Cartia also protected against blood clots and it was enteric coated, so I went with the Cartia option. The health benefits of garlic, ginger and turmeric were well known, but these I could simply obtain from a varied, nutritious diet. As it happened Peter and I are fond of Italian sauces and Indian curries.

Then there were the three drugs I'd been prescribed and/or recommended; viz. premia, ibuprofen and temazepam. The first two were no longer needed. However, I was bothered that I no longer slept as soundly as I would've liked. Dr Singh strongly advised against the drug temazepam, saying:

"No, don't take that drug. It's a benzodiazepine. You could easily become addicted. I have a better alternative. You should take melatonin as it's naturally produced by one's body."

As Dr Singh was writing out the prescription for Melatonin, which I was told I could get from my local compounding pharmacy, I remembered the prescription I'd received in late May from Dr Golledge. It was safely tucked in a zipped pocket of my handbag. When I produced it Dr Singh immediately exclaimed:

"You must take that drug. Go and get it before the script expires."

The drug voriconazole proved to be curative (see chapter 14), and I started taking it along with the four Complementary and Alternative Medicines (CAM). This initial treatment program took the best part of October, during which time Dr Singh recommended that I follow a very strict diet, consisting of:

"No sugar, dairy or wheat. Weekend treats only."

My lengthy consult was over, but I'd learnt an awful lot. Before leaving I unhesitatingly made a follow up appointment. Dr Singh's diagram illustrating the philosophy underlying his IM approach marked the start of more than a decade of support and invaluable advice and guidance.

Recognition of traditional healing methods

Dr Singh, trained in IM, wasn't alone in his broadminded approach to natural effective therapies. After all, in June and July thanks to a functional medicine doctor, my gut health had been restored. Dr Jenner the UK specialist had also recommended a holistic approach. Some of this terminology was new to me. It made me wonder if there were differences between the healthcare these doctors provided. Did they all provide equally effective therapies?

As I continued my investigations, I came across further healthcare systems. In May my sister had suggested acupuncture used by Traditional Chinese Medicine. Then there were all the Ancient Indian Traditions such as Ayurvedic Medicine. Exactly around the time I was looking for help that conventional Western Medicine didn't offer, none other than Dr Kerryn Phelps was calling for such traditional healing methods to be more widely recognised in my country. An article she wrote made me realise there was a global push for more recognition of worthwhile traditional healing approaches, particularly in the treatment of chronic disease like arthritis. As Dr Phelps was a past president of the Australian Medical Association (AMA), we had a high-profile trailblazer.

That weekend my attention was drawn to a book review in *The Australian* newspaper of a recent medical text that Dr Phelps and her colleagues had just published for general practitioners covering the integrative approach. There was no doubt in my mind that this book would contain answers to many of the questions I'd been confronted with.

However, the medical tome was expensive and besides it might have been filled with technical jargon beyond my comprehension. My best bet was to return to the Nedlands council library, even though it was highly unlikely they'd have such a book. The response I received from the librarians nearly blew me away. Unhesitatingly they did a catalogue search not just of the western suburbs library network, but also of the entire state of Western Australia. Sure enough a copy of Dr Phelps's book was located in a nearby hospital library. A request was placed on my behalf and within less than a week I was notified that it was ready to be collected. The text waiting on the reserved shelf for me was:

- Phelps, K. and others, 2011: *General practice; the integrative approach,* Elsevier, Sydney, Australia.

A medical text for GPs interested in an integrative approach

Once I'd returned home with the tome for GPs that had been entrusted to me, I immediately started scanning both contents and index looking for therapies that might alleviate and/or prevent further arthritic discomfort. To my delight I found OA was mentioned as a condition that could benefit from an integrative approach. Patients like myself were dissuaded from using drugs that could cause serious side-effects. Instead gentle exercise was suggested. In addition fish oil and even turmeric, an anti-inflammatory herb, were recommended.

There was also an entire chapter devoted to the relationship between the mind and body. Using medical but fairly easy to follow terminology, the impact that chronic stress could have on physical health was explained.

I realized that a text like the one Dr Phelps had produced could well help me identify other predisposing factors such as stress. For me a logical next step was to identify as many arthritis risk factors as I could that applied specifically to me.

The problem was I couldn't hold on to this informative text indefinitely. It would soon have to be returned to the hospital library. Ever the supporter of my wish to increase my understanding of those vicious attacks earlier in the year and their debilitating impact, Peter instantly ordered the thick volume. Imagine my delight when it appeared on the doorstep.

Flash-forward: IM now a part of Australia's mainstream medicine

In July 2021 Peter and I returned to have a philosophical chat with Dr Singh about the shifting sands in the body of medical wisdom. I also wished to clarify the terms holistic, functional medicine and Integrative Medicine.

At that stage I was midway through completing this book and Dr Singh had generously agreed to read the first draft. Even though I'd assured him that he was welcome to make corrections using a red pen if necessary, I found few changes had been made. However, he did point out that as the concept of Integrative Medicine (IM) is now recognised as mainstream in Australia, I should use capitals when referring to this recently accepted practice.

What had prompted the appointment was the diagram Dr Singh had drawn for me at my first meeting with him in September 2011; the one that had introduced me to the IM approach. A decade on and the label IM has come into use by the Australian Medical Association (AMA), to provide clarity as to what effective Integrative Medicine encompasses, as well as the philosophy underlying the modality.

As Peter and I walked out of the Claremont Medical Centre heading for home, my attention was drawn to the list of health services offered at the clinic. It made me catch hold of Peter's sleeve, because included under the list of general practitioners and specialists was the title Integrative Medicine. Together with IM were the services of a physiotherapist and a nutritionist.

Chapter 12 MY ARTHRITIS RISK FACTORS (Oct 2011)

Thanks to Dr Singh's belief in "empowering the patient through the use of an educational approach", I decided to put to use the knowledge I'd gained from medical texts together with advice from doctors. In May Dr Brennan, the gastroenterologist, had alluded to the role of the immune system. Since then doctors had hinted at other variables that may contribute to arthritis. All these pieces of information prompted me to start making a list. Would I be able to figure out the possible reasons underlying my susceptibility to arthritis?

By October 2011, a new mantra was in the forefront of my mind. I still believed that the saying "use it or lose it" had played a significant role in my recovery thus far, however I also feared a possible relapse. What I reminded myself was that "knowledge is power".

Possible factors that contributed to my arthritis (reviewed in 2021)

In 2021 with my book well underway, I leafed through a large lever-arch file of mine dated 2011. There among the lists of questions I'd asked Dr Singh was my first handwritten draft of Risk Factors. It amused me to see what I'd bravely written at the top of the A4 sheet of paper:

"How to fix arthritic knee and hip.

Step 1: Identify possible underlying causes and/or trigger factors.

Step 2: Address each factor and determine a solution."

At that point I didn't realise my notes, which stemmed from my usual logical and common-sense approach, would form the basis of a 'Personal List of Risk Factors.' My old handwritten draft had been annotated. Along with Dr Singh's neat ticks and suggestions was a new heading:

"Possible Arthritis Risk Factors".

The notes of our conversation from that appointment on October 18th 2011, suggested a hesitancy on my part. Probably I felt foolishly optimistic. Hence the question:

"Would it be silly of me ... even daft to attempt to prevent future attacks by addressing my list of risk factors?"

To which Dr Singh had given a positive and reassuring response. He'd firmly said:

"Not at all. I'm very impressed. If everyone did what you've done they would get better. You're not mentally ill."

Was Dr Singh being overly optimistic? Only time would tell.

Ten years on and I'm prepared to say he was correct. I did get better and I've remained well. Those April 2011 attacks weren't "ongoing" as had been predicted. Only one joint (my right hip) has been affected. Throbbing in my knee was resolved without any permanent damage being done. I continue to stride out, walking freely and easily. Chronic and degenerative prognoses haven't eventuated. My *arthritis* has remained in abeyance. I'm prepared to confidently state that with Dr Singh's help I was able to stop it.

I must concede though, that given the wisdom I've gained with hindsight and the advancements made by medical research, some adjustments to my 2011 Risk Factors have needed to be made. However, my reviewed 2021 personal list still exists as a reminder not to relax into complacency. Readers should also be made aware of the significant shift in medical knowledge that has occurred in the last decade. A causal risk factor for OA that was considered significant in 2011 by Modern Western Medicine has since been completely rejected. Today in Australia the "wear and tear" explanation is considered archaic (see chapter 27).

Back to 2011: Authoritative texts from Arthritis Foundation

In October 2011 Dr Phelps's tome for GPs had become my mainstay. It was my go to resource as I found her philosophy was in line with Dr Singh's; e.g. the significance of physical risk factors was recognised, but so too was the impact chronic stress could have on the body.

My collection of texts on arthritis continued to grow as on a visit to Western Australia's Arthritis Foundation centre, I spotted a glass-fronted cabinet containing resources for arthritis patients. Two volumes caught my eye:

- Lane, N.E. and others, 2002: *All about osteoarthritis; the definitive resource*, Oxford University Press, UK.

- Lam, P. and others, 2002: *Overcoming arthritis; a holistic plan to relieve pain and restore mobility,* Dorling Kindersley Pty Ltd, London, UK.

These texts, which Peter promptly ordered for me, were invaluable and brought me up to speed with medical thinking at that time. A new cause was being researched and one of my listed factors had been discarded. The "wear and tear" explanation for OA had been thrown out and some medical specialists were turning their attention to the role infections might play. Were bacteria causing the inflammations in arthritic conditions such as RA and ankylosing spondylitis?

So by the time I rewrote my arthritis risk factors in 2021 I'd formulated a clearer understanding of causal factors. These provided me with a plausible explanation for the events that had occurred in 2011. So it made sense to reorder my old list of factors; to correlate them with the sequence of sensations I'd experienced.

A hierarchy of causal factors

1. **Predisposing factor:** Genetic Marker (HLA-B27)

Back in 1997 I'd experienced an unpleasant sticky-feeling between my vertebrae towards the top of my spine, together with drumming discomfort in my wrists and feet (see chapter 4). In 2012 Dr Golledge ordered a test for the genetic marker linked to Ankylosing Spondylitis. It didn't surprise me to learn that it was positive.

2. **Basic causal factor:** Damaged Bowel

For 50 years of my life I lived with chronic constipation (see chapter 13). I was so used to it that I'd come to regard it as normal. In June 2011 the functional medicine doctor was the first to question me about bowel movements. In September 2011 Dr Singh reemphasized the importance of comfortable, daily elimination of waste.

3. **Fundamental factor:** Weakened immune system

Dysbiosis, an unhealthy ratio of pathogens to beneficial bacteria in the intestines can disturb the body's metabolism and weaken the immune system. *Prolonged stress can also cause spontaneous suppression of the immune response.* With a weakened immune system I was far more likely to develop infections.

4. **Subsequent factor:** Permeable intestines

Dysbiosis (Fungal/bacterial overgrowth) in the small intestine and colon can cause permeability and allow toxins etc. to enter the bloodstream. It's likely that an overload of toxins coupled with a weakened immune system left my body susceptible to infections.

5. **Resultant factor:** Infection

According to Dr Lam some arthritis specialists believe that bacterial infections may be the cause of inflammatory diseases like RA and Ankylosing Spondylitis. In September 2011 I was told that my joint had probably been damaged by an infection.

Dismissed and/or rejected factors:

Post-trauma arthritis can develop due to injury caused by a serious accident. However, I cannot remember any serious accidents that may have impacted on my hip. I believe the sudden, acute pain, together with ensuing throbbing, that I experienced in April/May 2011 was my body signaling an infection.

The "wear & tear" explanation I was given in April 2011 is now considered to be out of date. Dr Lane in her authoritative text clearly states that our joints are designed to last a lifetime. A study she discusses in her book shows that even the heavily used joints of marathon runners don't wear out. However, cartilage can be damaged by overuse if there has been previous joint injury.

Besides the adjustments I've made to my list due to current research regarding causal factors, I want to draw attention to the fact that the original heading on my handwritten note has also had to be modified. Quite simply I couldn't ultimately fix my right hip, even though for three years it felt fixed. But what's significant is that I did prevent my knee from being permanently damaged. The functional medicine doctor was absolutely correct when he stated:

"We can stabilise 'it', but we can't repair."

Treatments, interventions and lifestyle changes that worked for me

Thanks to my stubborn nature and dogged determination, together with serendipitous good fortune, all the causal factors underlying my arthritis were addressed.

The initial infection that marked the start of my problems was thankfully fairly promptly treated with macrodantin, an antibiotic which was really aimed at stopping a bladder infection. A year later in 2012, I received further extended antifungal treatment. During that therapy my thyroid and liver were closely monitored. This possibly indicated that hostile microorganisms had not only affected my right leg, but possibly also other organs.

The macrodantin antibiotic was an instant short-term solution as it immediately stopped the throbbing in my right leg. However, it was critically important that the source of the infection also be addressed. This required a three-pronged strategy. First the unhealthy dysbiosis in my gut had to be rectified. Here the functional medicine doctor played a key role. The second step required maintenance of my restored healthy gut-biome by following a diet rich in prebiotics and probiotics. At that stage in October 2011, my GP trained in Integrative Medicine stepped in with advice on a diet not unlike that of primitive hunters and gatherers. He told me that prebiotics and probiotics would assist in the repair of my mucosal intestinal barrier.

The third part of the strategy was to further reduce the risk of toxins leaking into my bloodstream. To ensure that the best possible conditions were provided for my colon to repair itself I made sure that, as far as daily bowel movements were concerned, it was smooth sailing. The gastroenterologist had suggested I use laxatives immediately to get things moving. Eventually I was pleased to find they became unnecessary. My new high fibre diet packed with unprocessed fresh fruit and vegetables took over and ensured regular action each morning.

The most important fundamental factor was the last to be concentrated on; viz. a weakened immune system. With my gut health restored I began to feel confident, but I was to learn that this still wasn't a complete solution. By taking a vitamin D supplement at breakfast I could further boost the function of my immune system, but stress levels also needed to be taken into account.

It hadn't been easy to steer my own course. At the beginning I'd appeared not to follow standard medical advice; e.g. corticosteroid injections weren't for me; fortuitously it turned out that antibiotics and an antifungal were a better alternative. It took courage to make decisions that weren't acceptable at the time. But thanks to the unwavering support of Peter and my broadminded GP I persisted. They provided reassurance and helped reduce stress levels.

Questions that remained unanswered

In spite of all the positive advances I'd made, I was still not satisfied. There were questions that I wished to find answers for, such as:

- Why had my left hip and leg remained unaffected?
- Why had my right leg throbbed and not my left?
- What was the underlying cause affecting my right hip?
- Why had Dr Brennan mentioned my immune system?

The gastroenterologist's parting comment continued to puzzle me. I recalled that in May I'd filed away his colonoscopy report without obtaining any further feedback from a GP. Fortunately, I remembered to take it with me when I returned to speak to the knowledgeable Integrative Medicine doctor.

Chapter 13 CHRONIC CONSTIPATION (Oct 2011)

Based on Dr Singh's positive response to my list of risk factors I knew that they had to hold some of the answers I sought. However, in October 2011 I hadn't yet worked out a hierarchical order of possible causes. I didn't fully understand the sequence of events that had brought about *'it'*. I asked myself whether my experiences in 1997 held a clue. When it comes to keeping track of my health I am orderly, possibly meticulous to a fault. This trait of mine, the one where I keep extensive records, continued to serve me well.

So my next list for Dr Singh documented significant ailments that I'd experienced dating back to 1992 when we'd lived on the crest of a hill in Mt Claremont, quite a distance from – and long before I knew about – the Whole Health Clinic in Hardy Road. Many of my new GP's patients had been seeing him for almost 40 years. In my case I needed to bring him up to speed and my briefly documented ailments did just that. After running his eye down my list he looked directly at me and said:

"I think you've had *'it'* twice. Tell me what happened in 1997".

As usual he was interested in getting the full picture, so he could more clearly understand how my mind and body responded to stress. My Notre Dame story, which I've summarised in chapter 4, elicited a decisive response. Unlike others, this doctor wasn't dismissive of Campbell's "cure". Instead, he promptly referred back to my list of risks and zeroed in on "Chronic/Lifelong Constipation".

It was Campbell's "cure" and my experience in 1997 that had led me to include constipation as an arthritis risk factor. When I'd followed his advice at the time and taken laxatives, my arthritic-like inflammation had soon cleared. This was not surprising as back then, more than 20 years ago, I didn't really know what constipation was. Peter and I actually used to joke about my ladylike "dassies". That was our code for my tiny, neat pellets, similar to those of a South African rock-rabbit or "dassie". I'd simply come to accept that the sparse droppings I produced were par for the course.

Fortunately, instead of ignoring the state of my bowel, Dr Singh was quite forthright and openly tackled the question.

"Do you have a bowel movement every day? ... Every day!" he emphatically emphasised.

"Yes", I sheepishly replied, too embarrassed to describe the appalling constipation which had dogged me since childhood. It was only thanks to Campbell's book that I'd come to realise that rock-hard, grape-like bunches of stool weren't actually normal. The concept of a daily BM stunned me. Most of the time I'd found it near impossible to dislodge the hard lumps which I could feel bulging up against the right side of my rectum.

Dr Singh was not satisfied. He probably read from my embarrassed expression that I was hiding something.

"What are they like? Are they like paste?"

"Yes," I again lied.

Then I mentioned that Dr Brennan, the gastro expert I'd seen in May, had encouraged me to use laxatives. Metamucil and Senokot had become a fixture on top of my spice rack in the kitchen.

An underlying cause for my constipation

Given Dr Singh's interest in the "Mind-Body" relationship, he pressed me with further questions as to why I'd developed severe constipation in 1997 and then again in 2010/2011.

"What was happening during those periods in your life? Were you particularly stressed?"

Given his kindly approach, I then confided in him, describing how the youngsters I worked with at Notre Dame University in 1997 had unkindly harassed me and that unreasonably high standards were expected; absolutely no mistakes tolerated. To add to this tension there had been no easily accessible toilets as the Catholic Church was in the process of converting old warehouses in the port city of Fremantle into university buildings. I'd also not plucked up the courage to ask for a brief tea-break during my long morning shift alone at the front desk. I confessed that my gut had shut-down for as long as 10 days at a time.

The 2010/2011 situation was different. During that December and January, Peter and I took a lengthy trip around the south island of New Zealand. All the travel had interfered with my bowel habits, which weren't great at the best of times. Without realising it my daily elimination of waste ground to a halt. My mind again played the same trick on my gut as it had done during my years as a librarian in Fremantle. Unconsciously I'd supressed the urge to poo.

During my appointment, Dr Singh had to address more than just my constipation issue, as by the end of October I'd completed the course of voriconazole prescribed by Dr Golledge. This specialist wished to review my response to his treatment.

Besides another referral to see the infectious disease expert, I was also given one to consult an endocrinologist. Dr Singh wanted to have my thyroid checked.

At the last minute I retrieved Dr Brennan's colonoscopy report from my handbag. As Dr Singh read the gastroenterologist's comments, I asked why only my right leg had throbbed and not my left.

There in the report was a vital clue. Dr Singh simply pointed to the phrase:

"Occasional diverticulum noted in the right colon – nil else noted." (see Figure 3).

On my return home I headed back to my downstairs study and impatiently searched my collection of arthritis texts. I'd been given a clue which I needed to follow up. The book that caught my eye was:

- Enders, G., 2014: *GUT; the inside story of our body's most underrated organ*, Scribe Publications, London, UK.

My sister Susan had given me the book for my birthday, but beyond a quick scan I'd not read the text in detail. Connections between disease and the gut were mentioned, but nothing about arthritis. This time I looked at the topics covered more closely. What I'd previously missed was Giulia Enders's coverage of the Bristol Stool Chart. This chart, developed by a doctor in Bristol in 1997, was a scale of 7 types of poo to illustrate what was ideal and what was unacceptable. It was a revelation as it confirmed why Dr Singh had emphasized a paste-like consistency. What was optimal was type 4, a sausage as smooth as toothpaste. Clearly this was an essential tool for an ignoramus like me as my constipation was off the chart. The medical term for my hard, grape-like mass of compacted lumps was faecal impaction; a very serious condition.

Giulia's book on the gut went on to explain that excessive pressure caused by hard stools could damage the bowel. Diverticula, or pouches were commonly created in the intestinal wall. Curiously I studied diagrams of a sigmoid colon with these pouches (see Figure 4).

A theoretical notion of mine

What if the excessive pressure I felt on my right side in my rectum, below the sigmoid colon, had caused a few tiny lesions or microscopic tears? Apparently microscopic lesions can occur anywhere in the GI tract and most of the time patients don't even know that they're there.

When I'd asked Dr Singh if a hostile microbe could move from the bowel into the body he'd replied in a matter of fact manner that,

"Yes, pathogens can escape into the body, but don't worry about it. You've got your immune system to keep a lid on them."

As an afterthought he added,

"Why don't you discuss this further with Dr Golledge. He probably knows about *'it'*, as his area of expertise is infectious disease."

The *'it'* conundrum

This *'it'* riddle continued to confront me, as did my intriguing arthritis puzzle. However, the more I persevered the more I discovered. There was no doubt in my mind that the functional medicine doctor knew his treatment was effective when he told me:

"We can stabilise *'it'*, but we can't repair." He'd added that he'd had *'it'*.

Dr Singh obviously believed in *'it'*, as I'd had *'it'* twice.

Now I learnt that Dr Golledge knew about *'it'*.

I was left wondering whether the well-known microbiologist would be able to explain *'it'* to me, and possibly even establish the link between hostile microbes and arthritis?

Chapter 14 DIAGNOSTIC TREATMENT (Nov 2011)

Towards the end of October 2011, I optimistically set off up Clifton Street towards the Hollywood Medical Centre where I'd first met Dr Golledge five months earlier. My sense of cheerful well-being stemmed from my achievements thanks to the therapies I'd received. The most recent of which was Dr Golledge's voriconazole. I'd started taking this antifungal on 26th September and had also begun the "hunter-gatherer diet" that he and my new GP had recommended. Dr Singh had summed up this diet by stating:

"No processed sugar, no dairy, no wheat. Weekend treats only."

On 4th October I'd got the full set of blood tests done which Dr Golledge had requested. I was hoping the results might reveal more to me about my mysterious 'it' condition. When I'd obtained my first box of voriconazole from the hospital pharmacy they'd provided me with several pages of information from Pfizer. True to form I'd diligently read it all. Points that drew my attention were: "Poor immune system" and "yeast infections". Maybe Dr Golledge would elaborate?

As I entered the smart reception area of the specialist centre I began to eagerly anticipate Dr Golledge's response to the progress I'd made. Confidently I thought that my problems were behind me. I didn't have to wait for long before I knew the answer.

With a broad smile this distinguished microbiologist greeted me. As we had quite a bit to discuss, he got straight down to business.

- *"So how have you been and how is your right leg? How well are you walking?"*

My demonstration took him by surprise, as I confidently stood up and raised my right foot, placing it against my left knee. Quietly I balanced, holding the position to the count of 10. Then I did the same thing with my left foot, while I stood stock still on my right; the once gammy leg. This was the last part of my exercise routine before I had my evening shower; my "piece de resistance".

- *"That's remarkable. In June I'd half thought you needed a THR done immediately. Have you been trying various additional therapies?"* Enthusiastically I told him all about the physio's dry-needling, the soothing, warm ultrasound therapy and my tailored home exercise program.
- *"Yes of course, you were keen to try alternative treatments. Remember I advised against taking ibuprofen long-term. Did you try complementary medications instead?"*

Well instead of starting voriconazole straight-away, I decided to act on a friend's suggestion and got my gut health restored first. She'd recommended her GP who was also a functional medicine doctor. He'd told me that I needed to address dysbiosis in my gut first, before commencing your treatment which would focus on the possibility that hostile toxins were impacting on tissues and organs beyond my gut.

- *Well now what I need to know is when did you complete the course of voriconazole that I gave you?*

Oh, I just finished it 4 days ago. I've also been following the "hunter-gatherer diet" you and Dr Singh recommended.

Dr Golledge was pleased to hear I'd taken his prescribed medication, but then it was my turn to ask a question:

"I don't fully understand why I've achieved success. Do you think I've put *'it'* all behind me?"

Dr Golledge replied kindly, saying:

"Well, your blood tests indicate that autoantibodies are attacking your thyroid. Other than that, I'm afraid we don't really know."

This news disappointed me because I felt I'd demonstrated that my troubles were behind me and that I was all good and ready to go. But instead he continued,

"Look you've shown a very positive response so I think it would be worth extending the voriconazole treatment.

In effect it will be diagnostic treatment and you never know we may be able to publish a paper discussing your case."

With that another prescription was written. Again it was for voriconazole, but this time the comprehensive treatment I'd begun in early October would continue for at least a further 10 months. This meant I'd be maintaining the "hunter-gatherer" low sugar diet, which included avoiding most processed foods, much like the diet of today's Hadza, an African "hunter-gatherer" tribe. It fascinated me to learn that these people are never obese but maintain a healthy weight throughout their adult lives. Of particular interest is the fact that their walking speed remains unchanged well into old age. To me this suggests that they don't suffer from arthritis.

This was what I needed to hear. Arthritis wasn't necessarily chronic and degenerative and it wasn't an old person's disease as many people think. It gave me the incentive to continue with a healthy diet for the rest of my life. What I've become used to eating more of are cruciferous veggies and leafy greens.

Both Dr Singh and Dr Golledge would monitor my progress throughout 2012 as I kept up monthly appointments, alternating between the two doctors. I couldn't have asked for better care and attention. But before I began the next lengthy phase of treatment I had to get my liver function tested. Both doctors wished to ensure that there was no sign of liver disease.

Well, Christmas fare that year would certainly be different, but come November I was relieved to be able to think of gift giving, rather than doctors' appointments. What remained to be scratched off my calendar was an appointment with an endocrinologist.

Chapter 15 MULTIDISCIPLINARY APPROACH (Nov 2011)

As 2011 drew to a close I came to fully appreciate why Dr Jenner had recommended in his book that arthritis patients would benefit from a multidisciplinary approach. By November I felt as though I'd consulted a bewildering array of health practitioners. Thankfully though, there were fewer cryptic responses and conflicting pieces of advice. I no longer felt it was necessary to seek second opinions. With my new considerate and well informed GP I had the support I needed. It was a relief not to have to make decisions on my own. Dr Singh took over the task of coordinating my healthcare with various specialists.

Referrals to a dermatologist & an endocrinologist

A chain of events in March 2011 had eventually led me to consulting an endocrinologist in November. I'd forgotten that the year had begun with a skin complaint; some kind of dermatitis that didn't respond readily to the creams that had been recommended. That was why I'd been referred to a dermatologist who unfortunately hadn't been particularly helpful. But in my usual determined fashion I'd not given up. Instead I'd asked to be referred to someone else. This was a good move as the second dermatologist had told me about "yeast infections". Along with a script for cream containing sulphur, he'd also requested blood tests to check my thyroid function. These tests went with a referral to see an endocrinologist at the Keogh Institute.

In April the blood tests had been completed, but then I'd been hit with those excruciating "arthritis attacks". Instead of visiting the

Keogh Research Institute up the road, I'd landed up seeing a radiologist, followed by Dr Brennan, the gastroenterologist.

Now the year was almost at an end and the referral to the endocrinologist still sat in my handbag's zipped pocket. When Dr Singh learnt about this he'd immediately encouraged me to make an appointment to see this specialist; a physician whose area of research was the endocrine system. My troublesome arthritic complaint which had started with changes on my skin, was apparently also linked to other conditions.

CAM: Complementary and alternative medications

In July/August my gut health had been restored, but now it had to be kept that way. To that point in time I'd largely followed the advice of health practitioners, including a functional medicine doctor and a physiotherapist. As a result the few purchases of vitamins and cod liver oil that I'd made at the Broadway health store in September had eventually expanded to a list of 10 items. The listed health benefits on the bottles often included "boosting the immune system", which was encouraging. However, the words "may help" (there was insufficient statistical evidence) created uncertainty. Still, it was reassuring that none of them at my low daily dose would be doing me harm.

Prior to my appointment at the Keogh clinic an envelope landed in my mailbox. Together with instructions on where to find the specialist's surgery, was a request that I make a list of all medications and supplements that I was taking. Instinctively I felt my list was too long, but what could be dispensed with? It was time for me to again visit the nutritionist at my Claremont Pharmacy.

As I sat down to chat with the nutritionist I told her as briefly as I could about all the successful therapies I'd received thanks to her initial guidance. A look of pleased satisfaction swept across her face when she learnt that I'd followed her advice and sought out doctors who knew about *'it'*. When I showed her the health program I was now on she quickly realised I'd covered everything. The "hunter-gatherer diet" supplemented with vitamins and minerals would ensure that I wasn't missing out on any essential nutrients. All that she suggested I add were a probiotic and a probiozyme which included digestive enzymes.

Appointment with an endocrinologist

Unlike the Harry Perkins Institute which was clearly visible at the end of Hampden Road, the Keogh Institute was buried within the depths of the Queen Elizabeth II Medical complex. I needed their detailed directions to find my way from our front door to the endocrine clinic.

The specialist I was to meet carried the title of Clinical Professor. This told me he would be at the cutting edge of medical knowledge involving the body's endocrine glands.

When my turn came to see Professor John Walsh he warmly greeted me as he invited me into his surgery. Immediately I felt comfortable with this softly spoken Englishman.

The professor had already familiarised himself with my blood test results, so he was able to immediately tell me that my thyroid was under attack. Even though it was still working, it was slowly being crippled. Apparently auto-antibodies that had been detected in my bloodstream, showed it was being damaged. He predicted that eventually it would stop working.

Ever the optimist I suggested that,

"Maybe an underlying cause could be found? If treated, couldn't the damage being done be reversed?"

To this he quietly replied,

"If your thyroid were to recover, I'd be very interested".

To complete his examination of my thyroid the doctor came to stand behind me while I remained seated. Very gently he palpated the central area of my neck. During this careful examination, he told me that besides my thyroid, the rest of my endocrine system was working well.

Before the end of the consultation I was relieved to learn he'd taken note of the vitamins and minerals I was taking. In particular he approved of the selenium Dr Singh had recommended. To ensure that I knew he wasn't suggesting something wacky, this professor went to the trouble of pulling out a couple of recently published research papers. One was from Germany and one from Japan. As it happened, I was quite happy to take him at his word.

His parting comment was very reassuring:

"You are well and at the moment I have no concerns. Your adrenal glands are working well and show no signs of depletion. Your thyroid is also functioning normally, but I will recommend that your GP be aware you're at risk of developing hypothyroidism."

With that I was given another request for thyroid function tests. The results would be sent to Dr Singh.

My Updated Preventative Treatment Plan

Back to my GP's Whole Health Clinic I went, eager to learn the results of my thyroid tests.

As I sat down alongside Dr Singh's desk I couldn't help but notice a report from Professor Walsh in front of him. He'd just read it and was keen to share the good news.

"Your thyroid function is good. Dr Walsh has noted that the treatment regimen you outlined has dramatically improved your health.

He's also recommended you include selenium supplementation at a dosage of 200ug daily."

At that point I was glad Dr Singh was so thorough and knowledgeable about complementary and alternative medications. He knew that selenium could be toxic in high doses, so he wanted to closely check my list of vitamins and minerals. It turned out that one of the preparations also contained selenium.

When he told me this, I mentioned that I'd begun including brazil nuts in my diet. They'd been listed in Jenkins's book as "a very good source of selenium". Dr Phelps had also given selenium a tick of approval as it had been shown to boost the immune system.

Dr Singh being a well-informed IM doctor, then told me garlic was another good food source of selenium. Maybe I was in danger of taking too high a dose?

Obviously, my treatment plan needed to be consolidated. By the time my appointment was over the list of supplements had been almost halved in number. Certain key vitamins remained, and I continue to take them to this day. In fact vitamin D3 hit the headlines when the COVID pandemic struck in 2020. It's now known that vitamin D3 can play an important prophylactic role in preventing and/or weakening infections.

The last items my GP turned his attention to were the prebiotic and probiozyme capsules. He wanted me to replace them with,

"lactose free acidophilus powder,"

And emphasised that,

"your breakfast yoghurt isn't enough!"

"Now, before the end of the year I'd like you to see Dr Greg Witherow; an orthopaedic surgeon".

I felt a bit disappointed as the way in which my health was steadily improving left me feeling confident that the holistic treatments were working. I felt well and I was walking well. Maybe I could legitimately postpone the hip replacement that some doctors thought would be needed sooner rather than later? However, Dr Singh cautioned me not to be too optimistic. My treatment couldn't be regarded as foolproof. Doctors had to collect a lot of positive evidence for a treatment to be recognised as statistically significant.

Remaining unanswered questions

With insufficient medical data there was no clear-cut evidence as to whether my preventative treatment & supplements would continue to work. Essentially, I'd decided to be a guinea pig, or lab rat if you will. I would wait 10 years before finding answers to these questions:

- Would a healthy diet based largely on whole, fresh food restore daily, smooth BMs?
- Would a healthy gut biome facilitate repair of my intestinal lining?
- Would the "arthritis attacks" recur, or had they been stopped?
- Would I remain free from all arthritic pain and discomfort?
- Would I continue to walk briskly ... even run?
- Would all joints other than my right hip remain in good condition?
- Would my left hip joint continue to show no signs of "wear & tear"?

Only time would tell.

Chapter 16 NO IMMINENT HIP SURGERY (Dec 2011)

It turned out that Dr Witherow's skills were in high demand. The only appointment available was a cancellation towards the end of November. Five days before my appointment with him I was to get my right hip X-rayed for the third time that year.

At that stage it was natural for me to wish to avoid, or at the very least postpone major hip surgery as I was no longer experiencing any pain, or discomfort of any sort. Furthermore, I'd been alerted to a significant event which was occurring at the time in Sydney's law-courts. This information emphasised the need for me to proceed with caution.

Total hip replacement (THR) lawsuits

Just prior to my appointment with Dr Witherow, another serendipitous moment occurred. It was almost as though I had a guardian angel at my shoulder.

My husband and I were invited out to dinner by Jim, a former inter-state colleague. The two men had become close friends over the years and often caught up for a casual lunch. However, on that occasion his wife was with him, so an opportunity was created for me to meet her. It was a chance encounter, but it was providential.

Jim's wife Irene was a trained nurse who worked for an international supplier of medical prosthetics. Knowing this, it didn't take long before I got around to talking about the hip replacement decision I faced. A round table discussion began and what this well-informed couple had to tell me made my jaw drop.

Apparently, Irene's father had just undergone THR surgery. What horrified me was that the same procedure had been redone three times in five years. Her Dad's hip prosthetic had been repeatedly replaced and as a result he could no longer walk properly.

The round table discussion that ensued raised the question as to why this medical debacle had occurred. I was all ears, as here were people relating a recent awful experience, but they also could add significant background information. I needed to hear this in order to help me make another very significant decision.

Right at that time a test case was going through the Sydney law courts. THR patients who'd become wheelchair bound were suing a company and what was being contested were "dodgy cobalt joints". As often occurs in such cases, the company lawyers were looking for someone else to blame. They were saying that the surgeons were at fault for not fitting the prosthetics properly. They were alleging that this was the reason why metal-on-metal joints were wearing badly and poisoning people's systems with filaments. Irene's father had also been told there were "problems with the glue!"

This nonsense was unlikely to stand up in court in Australia, as in the UK a hip replacement recall had already been issued. Then there was the US. Almost 10,000 hip replacement lawsuits were pending in Texas.

This stunning information was followed with another story which left me feeling uneasy. Sadly Jim and Irene had a close friend who suffered from leukaemia. Following chemotherapy he'd been left disabled as fungal infections had damaged two of his joints; his knee and his elbow.

These bad news stories left me bewildered. This was a lot of information to process before my appointment with Dr Greg Witherow, an orthopaedic surgeon who would exceed my expectations.

My individualised health strategy

Given the encouragement and advice I'd obtained from the medical texts written by Dr Campbell, Dr Jenner and Dr Phelps, together with Dr Singh's belief in empowering the patient, I'd formulated my own health strategy. This strategy, which aimed at *"driving arthritis into complete remission"*, consisted of 3 parts:

1. <u>My Pain/Discomfort and Mobility Record</u>

My record covering all arthritic sensations and the associated restrictions to movement; viz.

PAIN, ranging from excruciating, acute pain to unpleasant tingling (paraesthesia).

MOBILITY RESTRICTIONS, ranging from a peg-leg gait to minimal restriction in range of motion.

2. <u>My Risk Factors</u>

Features that predisposed me to an arthritic condition; i.e. information relating to my condition that I collated from GPs' & specialists' tests & advice, medical texts and research papers.

3. <u>My Personal Treatment Regimen</u>

Healthy eating, based largely on a "Hunter & Gatherer's diet" and supplemented with vitamins, minerals, probiotics, a probiozyme capsule and fish oil; i.e. a treatment program based on advice amalgamated from a number of health care providers.

This health program that I'd devised by amalgamating advice from the health care providers I consulted, had been remarkably successful. By November my gammy right leg had recovered; regained strength and full range of motion. I was also entirely free of any pain or discomfort. For these reasons I'd begun to question earlier medical advice; viz. "You need hip surgery". So, before my appointment I put together the 3 documents I had created. I hoped that these records would encourage Dr Witherow to adopt a conservative approach to treatment.

Appointment with the orthopaedic surgeon

It wasn't surprising that Dr Witherow was exceedingly busy given the number of cases to be dealt with before the Christmas holiday season. Nevertheless, he couldn't have been nicer, as he took time to show me my X-rays and to point out key features such as the large cyst and labral tear. An assessment of my range of motion followed and as I popped myself up onto the examination table, I was able to demonstrate how agile I was. The surgeon didn't comment, but as I quietly lay flat on my back he simply asked:

"Can you touch your toes?"

That task was easily accomplished thanks to the dry-needling therapy I'd received. Then came a response from Dr Witherow which made me smile:

"I don't think an operation is indicated".

With that he excused himself as he had another patient waiting. Fortunately, I wasn't left with unanswered questions as a visiting trainee surgeon from the UK took over.

This doctor was on a fellowship program so she had more time to spend with me. I was able to show her my pain records, risk factors and treatment regimen. She was intrigued and asked if she could make copies for herself. On her return from the photocopier I again asked the question:

"Could an infection move from the bowel to the hip?"

Her response matched the advice I'd obtained from the US doctor earlier in the year (referred to in chapter 2). She readily admitted that it was possible for the bowel to be a source of infections. She went on to confirm the previous advice I'd received from the other side of the world, saying:

"Normally we would've tested the synovial fluid in your hip joint, but now there's no point because you've started a course of voriconazole."

With that she handed me a copy of a paper published by the Arthroplasty Society of Australia. It advised that patients be given antibiotics prior to surgery if they had infective problems such as dental issues. This suggested a rotten tooth could also land up affecting a hip joint.

Given the active interest I'd demonstrated and the efforts I'd made to help myself, this lovely doctor then offered to send me a personal copy of the surgeon's report which my GP would be receiving.

As I left and made my way down the passage towards the receptionist's front desk, I sensed that I was being watched. Glancing over my right shoulder I noticed the two surgeons I'd just met were observing my progress. I suspect they couldn't believe their eyes. With a brief wave I confidently continued along the corridor "walking freely and easily".

Sound reasons for my deferring hip surgery

No longer did I feel utterly perplexed by *'it'*, but I did remain uncertain; unsure that I had made the right decision. Was surgery still needed? Was it foolhardy of me to postpone the operation? Was I in denial; unable to face the inevitable?

Within less than a week I received a reassuring answer. Dr Witherow's report landed in my mailbox. It gave me the feedback I sought:

- "the repeat MRI shows moderately severe OA of her hip joint"
- "an infection has affected her hip and, potentially, other areas"
- "range of motion in her hip is markedly improved"

He summed up these findings with the statement:

- "I don't believe an operation is indicated as she is asymptomatic and there's an ongoing infective problem."

An informative response such as this was just what I needed. My confidence was boosted knowing I'd made the right decision to delay surgery. More pieces of my arthritis puzzle were starting to fall into place. Glimmerings of light appeared as to what *'it'* was. What was of particular significance was the reference to an "ongoing infective problem", and the mention of "potentially other areas".

Chapter 17 MIND-BODY STRESS REDUCTION (Dec 2011)

When November 2011 ended I was on cloud nine, secure in the knowledge that I'd found an experienced surgeon who was in no hurry to recommend surgery. He would wait until I was ready to make such a major decision; until I knew without a shadow of a doubt that it was necessary. To my surprise and to the surprise of many doctors, a number of years passed before I considered going under the knife.

So it was a pity that my ebullience lasted less than a week. Shortly after my appointment with Dr Witherow, I received a scary phone call and if that wasn't enough Peter was startled one morning by what he spotted on my lower back.

"Other areas" affected

When I heard Dr Singh's voice on the other end of the phone I'd cheerily responded, eager to tell him that surgery wasn't imminent. But my doctor was in no mood to chat, instead there was a sense of urgency as I was told in no uncertain terms to:

"Stop taking voriconazole immediately! You will be hearing from Dr Golledge shortly."

So why had I received that urgent phone call about voriconazole?

It was because the November liver function tests indicated,

"an acute hepatitis picture."

My liver had become seriously inflamed. It wasn't in as robust good health as they'd thought. This was contrary to what the recent tests for liver disease had indicated.

My treatment was abruptly suspended; further blood tests and doctors' appointments postponed. I was to make a follow-up appointment in mid-January.

This news came out of left field. None the wiser, I simply turned my attention to Christmas preparations. But within days Peter spotted something significant on my lower back. It was early one Sunday morning, so there'd been no breakfast rush before work, I hadn't even finished getting dressed. Wearing only my favoured white, cotton undies I was in the midst of a vigorous teeth-brushing session when an exclamation from Peter startled me.

"What's that on your back?"

Had he spotted a creepy crawly? I hadn't felt anything, so I simply responded:

"There's nothing."

"No ... look ... turn around. Can you see in the mirror?"

I needed my hand-mirror in order to obtain a clear view of the lower part of my back. What was reflected in the mirror made me shudder slightly. I didn't like what I saw as it looked as though I'd been scratched, not once but twice. Close to my "dimples of venus" (shallow symmetrical indentations) and equidistant from my spine were two distinct and practically, identical scrape-marks, a bit like lesions. Their appearance was identical, suggesting they were linked to a part of my anatomy.

We were stunned, but relieved that I felt no discomfort. What made us curious was that the two marks were so similar in appearance and location. Did those patches indicate that something may well have escaped into my body? After all such a possibility had been suggested.

Ever curious I wondered about this strange phenomenon. Then I recalled that I knew of an infective agent that behaved in such a manner. It was the chicken pox virus ... once it's invaded our body it never leaves. Instead in a sinister fashion it latches onto parts of our nervous system and lurks there patiently waiting for an opportunity to emerge and strike out at its host. In fact I remember witnessing such an attack. My brother once suffered through shingles which covered only the left side of his face.

Had something, possibly a virus, latched onto my nervous system?

Traditional Chinese Acupuncture

The liver scare together with the shocking surprise of two mysterious lesions on my lower back were an alarming setback. I felt as though I was in a state of limbo as my doctors wouldn't consider continuing treatment until they were sure my liver had recovered. It was all rather unsettling.

Feeling a bit at a loss, I turned my attention to finding some additional support. As my stock of vitamins, in particular vitamin D, was running low, I headed back to my local health food store the next morning. Of course, in the back of my mind was the thought that I'd again have an opportunity to discuss my health issues with someone. Maybe the young man who'd enthused about Dr Singh would provide some more helpful ideas.

I was not disappointed. Young Alex readily suggested I explore what Traditional Chinese Medicine had to offer. He gave me the title of a book which he'd found informative:

- Beinfield, H. and Korngold, E., 1991: *Between heaven and earth. A guide to Chinese medicine,* Random House, New York, USA.

Then he told me about the Arthritis Foundation in Shenton Park, which had a bookstore. It was there that I found a helpful book written by a medical doctor who'd emigrated from China with his parents when he was young.

- Lam, P. and others, 2002: *Overcoming arthritis; a holistic plan to relieve pain and restore mobility,* Dorling Kindersley Pty Ltd, London, UK.

Dr Paul Lam now lived in Sydney where he practiced as a family physician. Why his book attracted my attention was that he'd been diagnosed with arthritis in his twenties. Instead of simply accepting the diagnosis which included taking arthritis drugs for the rest of his life, he'd explored alternatives. Given his heritage these naturally included Traditional Chinese Medicine.

Both these texts discussed the ancient art of Chinese acupuncture dating back thousands of years. What struck me was the difference between this traditional therapy and the dry-needling technique the physiotherapist had used. Both methods used fine needles, but not in the same way. The dry-needling I'd received in September had released tension in taut and knotted muscles and successfully removed residual arthritic discomfort. Come December I needed a different treatment.

I was emotionally tense and perturbed by those lesions that looked like scratch marks on my back. Apparently traditional acupuncture had a calming effect as the fine needles released stress-relieving endorphins. Where would I find a practitioner of such calming, feel-good treatment?

I recalled having been told earlier in the year about a healer who practiced this particular, traditional form of acupuncture (see chapter 6). I knew his clinic was nearby in Dalkeith. A quick search for this healer's website helped me easily decide on my next course of action. What he offered in conjunction with acupuncture was a stress-reduction programme.

Mind-body stress-reduction treatment

The blue house on the corner was hard to miss. As I approached the front door, I noticed a small sign poking out of the lawn. All that was written on it was "acupuncture"; no elaboration appeared necessary. There was another patient quietly waiting his turn, so with some time on my hands I decided to read the noticeboard. Pasted there were newspaper cuttings from The West Australian. The articles trumpeted the Chinese practitioner's achievements. It was all very encouraging.

Once I'd sat down, the other patient spoke up. He must've recognised that I was a newcomer as he wished to reassure me by relating his own positive experience. I was to discover that this doctor, who'd studied Traditional Chinese Medicine (TCM), was highly regarded. In his homeland he carried the title of Professor. Apparently, his acupuncture skills were even recognised in Australia. It surprised me to learn that I could make a legitimate claim for his treatment from my private health fund.

When my turn came to receive treatment the first thing that struck me was the pleasant aroma that wafted through the door as I entered. It might have been lavender, or maybe another aromatic herb that I wasn't familiar with.

Much like the physiotherapist's consulting room there was a massage table which occupied most of the space. Before I lay down the Chinese healer asked me a few questions. I didn't go into extensive detail but simply mentioned the key issues; viz. my gut and hip. Then I realised what was really bothering me at the time were those "scratch-like lesions" close to my "dimples of venus", so I asked whether he could give me his opinion as to what they might be. With that my pulse and tongue were checked, followed by an examination of those "scratches". Little was said other than the brief comment:

"They're on your kidney meridians."

Soon the stress-reduction programme was underway. Initially I was a bit tense as I anticipated feeling sharp twinges from the fine needles. But I had nothing to fear. I barely felt a thing; all I heard was the quiet murmur:

"Relax ... just relax."

The treatment was so soothing that before long I sensed myself nodding off.

Shortly before Christmas with the programme completed, I was simply told,

"Your mind and body are now in balance."

There's no doubt I'd benefitted from the healer's support, as I truly felt a sense of emotional and physical well-being. Those "scratch-like lesions" had also vanished which was a relief.

As with the IM approach, this healer regarded the body as a whole. The mind influenced the body and likewise the body could impact on the mind. Well, I'd come around to recognising in 2011 that my mind could certainly play tricks on my gut. There'd been times in my life when it had barely functioned.

Christmas was an enjoyable distraction, but I was impatient and wished my next appointment with Dr Singh hadn't been delayed until January. I knew I needed to find out more about the mind-body connection and how it could impact on the immune system. Could it also play a major role in staving off my arthritis?

Chapter 18 WHOLE PERSON CARE (Jan 2012)

The feeling of physical wellbeing that I felt after the TCM healer's stress-reduction programme wasn't momentary; it was significant. While I waited for my next appointment with Dr Singh, my GP, I decided to find out more about mind-body medicine. An entire chapter in the book by Dr Phelps discussed this topic in depth. The role that chronic stress played in the disease process was emphasised.

The effect of stress

Dr Brennan, the gastroenterologist, had previously alerted me to the possibility that the immune system could be a factor contributing to my arthritis (see chapter 5). By the end of that year my positive response to antibiotic treatment strongly suggested an "infective problem". If my immune system had been weakened it wouldn't be properly doing its job of protecting me from harmful invaders that caused inflammation and infection.

I later discovered that prolonged stress could have weakened my immune system. This was why I'd mentioned it in relation to my arthritis risk factors. Of the five factors I'd identified (see chapter 12), my GP had zeroed in on the impact of chronic stress and the role it played in contributing to illness.

As Dr Phelps's book was directed at those with medical training, all the biological processes caused by an extended fight-or-flight response were discussed in technical terms. However, I could understand that an excess of stress hormones like adrenaline and cortisol weren't good for me in the long run. If stressors weren't dealt with, my digestive system and my immune system could stop working properly, thus heightening the chance of infections. Apparently, there's increasing evidence that this can indeed contribute to arthritis flares; i.e. the episodes of inflammation and/or infection that I'd experienced.

Impact of Central Nervous System on Digestive System (Gut), Immune System & Endocrine System

My personal health strategy had begun with my digestive system and the problem of chronic constipation. Once that function had been restored to good, working order (see chapters 8 & 13), I'd turned my attention to appropriate ways of viewing and dealing with stressors. Consequently, I hoped that my immune system had been bolstered. Fortunately, this appeared to be the case as there were no longer any signs of arthritic inflammation and/or infection.

Stress had impacted on my brain and central nervous system, which then had had a knock-on effect and impaired my immune system. Now I was to learn of another system that was also interrelated. To my surprise it was my endocrine system (see Figure 7).

In November 2011 the endocrinologist I'd consulted had requested blood tests to detect thyroid disease. Dr Singh had then requested further blood tests for thyroid issues & autoantibodies (TSH, TPO AB TgAb), my liver function, vitamin D and cholesterol levels. Besides this usual list he'd added a range of tests for other ailments caused by viruses. Clearly, he wasn't going to leave any stones unturned.

The results were to be reviewed at my next appointment in the following January.

January 2012 appointment with my GP trained in Integrative Medicine

When I returned to Dr Singh in early January 2012, I was to learn more about the whole person approach and the impact of stress. More information was also provided about the various biological sub-systems that function in unison and keep our bodies in good working order.

As usual my GP's advice and support were invaluable. Not only did he spend time explaining the many variables involved. He also used diagrams to illustrate the impact that stress can have on the body. In conclusion he emphasised that the many biological systems in our bodies are all interconnected.

As Dr Singh knew which associations to look for, he wasn't surprised to find the blood test results confirmed that I'd had a past infection with the common Epstein-Barr virus. What interested me was to learn that,

"EBV has been associated with thyroiditis."

The next bit of feedback was very encouraging as in June 2011 the blood tests requested by a dermatologist had recorded an exponential climb in thyroid autoantibodies. Now I was told:

"The upward trend in autoantibodies has been reversed and your cholesterol level is also coming down."

My sluggish thyroid had started to recover and my cholesterol level didn't require immediate attention. As an under-functioning thyroid is strongly associated with unhealthy cholesterol levels, it wasn't surprising that an improvement in my thyroid function had resulted in lower cholesterol levels.

Dr Singh was also relieved to report that,

"Your liver function is returning to normal, but it isn't yet within an acceptable range."

I would have to patiently wait until my next appointment with Dr Golledge, the infectious disease specialist who'd taken charge of my case. Hopefully he'd agree to resuming the beneficial voriconazole treatment.

My Concept of *'it'*

Before the end of my appointment, Dr Singh added another diagram to his "Stress impact" chart. In addition to explaining stress and the mind-body connection, he drew attention to 3 interconnected biological systems that applied to my thyroiditis; viz.

- Central Nervous System – Immune System – Endocrine System.

He even went further and suggested a possible link between the Epstein-Barr virus and the thyroid.

So, was EBV the mystery *'it'* I wondered?

Dr Singh then explained to me that *'it'* wasn't a specific pathogen, but rather a <u>concept or theory that involved infective agents.</u> It was a complex condition that doctors didn't fully understand. This concept was still considered a bit controversial, so it wasn't covered in medical textbooks. But medical researchers had started to uncover links between infective agents, autoimmune disease and the gut.

By that stage I'd used up my allotted time. Other patients were waiting and I realised how fortunate I was to be able to anticipate obtaining more feedback the following month from Dr Golledge, the clinical microbiologist.

Chapter 19 TEAM MANAGEMENT (Jan – Dec 2012)

The year 2012 was a very good one ... I got better and better. My leg continued to strengthen and as I felt no discomfort, I started to forget the agonising pain I'd experienced in May 2011. Medical treatment was more straightforward too. Instead of a series of referrals to quite a number of specialists, a team management approach was adopted. Two doctors took me under their wing; a clinical microbiologist and a GP trained in integrative medicine.

Both Dr Golledge and Dr Singh were interested in my case. They knew about *'it'* which involved my immune system and probably an infective agent of some sort. What I'd begun to realise was that my complex condition, which had forcefully announced its presence in the previous May, had had a more widespread impact other than my uncomfortably sore right leg.

Throughout 2011 my doctors and I had followed a trail of clues or ailments:

- Skin issues; e.g. eczema patches near right hip & behind right knee
- Pain in right leg; e.g. excruciating acute episode & throbbing knee
- Thyroid problem; i.e. presence of autoantibodies
- Liver inflammation
- Scratch-like lesions on "kidney meridians"

In 2012 I continued my quest which was to develop some sort of understanding of this complex condition that involved my whole body. My aim was to increasingly come to grips with how and why I had to boost my immune system.

Voriconazole treatment resumed

By the end of November 2011 I'd completed my first course of voriconazole. Dr Golledge had started me on quite a strong dose of 400mg daily, as my blood tests hadn't revealed any sign that my liver function might be compromised. Everything had gone without a hitch as far as I was concerned. Other than the minor glitch of "scratch-marks" appearing on my lower back, I'd suffered no adverse side-effects. The urgent phone call from my GP instructing me to stop taking the medication immediately, had come out of the blue (see chapter 17).

Fortunately my liver had immediately shown signs of recovery, so when I next spoke to Dr Golledge I was hoping to learn that my liver function had bounced back and was again in good nick. As far as I was concerned my liver function was a side issue. My focus was on my weak right leg which I was aiming to fully restore to normal. For these reasons my response to Dr Golledge's opening question was probably inappropriate. When he asked:

"So how have you been?"

I was unsure how to respond. After all I felt absolutely fine, so instead of talking I decided a quick demonstration would be the go.

At a previous appointment I'd gaily balanced on one leg; first my right and then my left. This time I decided to do one better by raising my right leg high to show how easily I could step over a knee-high wall into our shower. At the same time I explained that 10 months ago this was beyond me; getting into our shower was a struggle.

To this he simply nodded and I realised that my agility wasn't his primary concern, as he then went on to say my liver was rapidly improving.

"At this rate we can resume voriconazole treatment, but at a lower dose of 100mg daily."

Extensive blood tests covering thyroid, liver and kidney functions

Again I'd been handed another blood test request form. It was quite an extensive list covering thyroid, liver and kidney functions. It was also reassuring that signs of inflammation would be looked for. I knew from my background reading that any evidence my liver was under attack from a virus would be swiftly picked up.

The next time I visited Dr Singh's surgery marked the start of an exciting health journey. Everything was looking good. However, my doctors adopted a cautious approach and resumed treatment with a low 100mg dose of voriconazole. Given my GP's knowledge of complementary medications he also gave me the name of a herbal product: Milk Thistle, or to be precise the active ingredient "silymarin", which is known to have anti-inflammatory properties. This herb would help protect my liver and I was pleased to learn from him that its traditionally known benefits were now being proven by scientific research.

Given all my results were so positive, I asked my GP if he would provide me with copies of them. I was eager to share these positive results with Peter, whom I knew would be keenly interested.

Indeed Peter was fascinated and so was I. We were amazed by the number of results listed. Records of both liver and thyroid function had been kept stretching back to June of the previous year. We could see why the markers for liver inflammation were highlighted in red; they were very high. Fortunately, the rapid recovery rate was also apparent.

Graph of TSH (Thyroid Stimulating Hormone) levels

It was the thyroid results that initially grabbed our attention. TSH, the "thyroid stimulating hormone", was the marker used to indicate thyroid function. I pointed to the levels in early June and July 2011. In less than a month there'd been a 45% increase in TSH levels from 2.87 to 4.15. What had caused this sudden spike, I wondered? Had I felt anything around that time? Of course, there had been a significant event in May 2011 when I'd experienced a major, excruciating attack; an inflammation/infective episode.

With this link to what had occurred in May 2011, I hoped to be able to: address my risk factors (see chapter 12), and make the necessary lifestyle changes; i.e.

"use primary prevention to keep those excruciating and damaging attacks at bay."

I resolved to continue my quest to develop a plausible, overall understanding of what had occurred. The blood test results weren't filed away and forgotten, but instead our graph of TSH levels would extend over 4 years, beginning in June 2011 and ending in July 2015. Eventually, the slow rise in TSH levels following the end of voriconazole treatment couldn't be ignored. I'd managed to briefly reverse the trend for 6 months by secretly self-medicating with a 50mg daily dose of voriconazole. But once the few voriconazole (Vfend) tablets that I still had were used up, the gradual TSH rise continued (see Figure 5).

Extraordinary Liver Function results from voriconazole treatment

The absence of a clear-cut explanation for why TSH levels had sharply risen in June 2011 and then suddenly reversed their upward spike, didn't deter Peter and me. We decided to also plot the ALT results indicating liver function. They also began in June 2011 and had revealed the "hepatitis picture" that occurred in November 2011.

Alarmed, my doctors had told me to immediately stop treatment. My liver had then very rapidly recovered and I had resumed the medication towards the end of January at a low 100mg daily dose. So confident was Dr Golledge in his treatment that he gradually increased this dose from 100mg to 300mg in small 50mg increments. Surprisingly there was no adverse inflammatory reaction. In fact the opposite occurred; the higher the dose, the more positively my liver responded. Without a doubt it was doing my liver good.

By August the blood test results for liver and thyroid had returned to normal. My test results were hugely rewarding as they showed a list of numbers in "black", TSH included. Thyroid autoantibodies were still a bit high, but even they were drifting down.

But what voriconazole had done for me and my liver was truly impressive, particularly as it was counter-intuitive. You see, over the previous 6 months as Dr Golledge had slowly but surely increased the dose from 100mg to 300mg, no "acute hepatitis picture" had appeared. Unlike what had occurred in November 2011, my response was positive; i.e. the higher the dose, the more my liver had improved. About a year later in January 2014 an ALT level of 13 showed my liver continued to function healthily; well within the normal 7 to 35 range.

These findings made me wonder whether the voriconazole treatment could have eradicated a toxin from my liver. This notion felt a bit fantastical, so I quietly kept such ideas to myself. Instead I was simply grateful that Dr Golledge had been prepared to give it his best shot (see Figure 6).

The end of voriconazole treatment

The way my body responded to treatment during 2012 had been extraordinary. My liver, my thyroid and my right leg returned to good working order. At that stage I even started to entertain the notion that instead of "degenerating cartilage" maybe mine was repairing itself.

But in October 2012 Dr Golledge discounted and corrected such fanciful notions. Apparently, cartilage could only recover in a petri dish as it didn't contain nerves and blood vessels; once severely damaged it would steadily erode with use. It interested me to learn that doctors could actually grow cartilage in petri dishes and then even replace cartilage in some patients, rather than carrying out a total hip replacement. But they only did this for the young. At close to 60 years I was too old, besides cartilage replacement required at least 4 months of complete bed rest. Given this background, he gently but firmly said,

"No, we wouldn't do that to you."

Instead he gave me a referral for another MRI of my right hip. I optimistically still hoped there'd be signs of improvement as I felt absolutely no discomfort or pain. The comment from Dr Golledge's report that my GP read to me later that month indicated the doctors were still in disbelief:

"As you know Mary Anne remains well and continues to confound us."

Conclusion

At the end of 2012 before Dr Golledge started reviewing my final test results for the year, I heard a barely audible mutter:

"Ah ... pity ... it's got your thyroid."

'It' would remain an unidentified culprit.

But then he quickly shrugged off the disappointment and resumed his usual upbeat stance; saying,

"Look, your thyroid function has improved, but eventually you'll develop Hashimoto's hypothyroidism."

He went on to add, "Your MRI does show you're not having much luck regenerating cartilage. But if you're not in any pain you don't have to go back to see Dr Witherow."

Both pieces of news were a bit disheartening, and it probably showed on my face, so to cheer me up he continued by saying,

"Look, you are feeling well and you look very well. You must be doing something right. Don't worry, your immune system is now firing on all cylinders."

It was Dr Singh who gave me the extra reassurance I needed. At my last appointment for the year he gave me more feedback and clarified my understanding of what the voriconazole had achieved. Basically the antifungal treatment had given me a reprieve. He told me with a broad smile that I shouldn't be worried as,

"You've got your immune system. It will look after you."

By December 2012 my immune system had apparently been strengthened and could fight my battles for me. Both doctors had told me that with a robust immune response I could go forward, confident in the knowledge that my body would help me resist future infections

Chapter 20 AN INFECTIVE PROBLEM (Apr 2013)

Once the voriconazole treatment had been completed there was no longer any further need for team management. Opportunities to ask Dr Golledge for further explanations came to an end. But what I did have were my graphs recording changes in both thyroid and liver function. I decided to use these objective blood test results to develop my understanding of what might have happened in May 2011 and throughout 2012. For my own peace of mind I needed to clarify this concept.

My Concept (My theoretical understanding)

Peter continued to serve as my sounding board. The ideas that I outlined to him were largely based on feedback from the doctors and specialists I'd consulted over the previous 18 months. In simple terms this is what I'd grasped at that point:

The first part of <u>My Concept</u> considers the possibility that prolonged, undue tension may result in a weakened immune response. This idea involves 4 key systems in our bodies; viz.

- the central nervous system
- endocrine system
- circulatory system
- immune system & the Gut

It's our bloodstream, together with other parts of the circulatory system, that interconnects these biological units in our body. If a patient experiences undue and prolonged tension it can interfere with the normal, healthy role of these systems.

Peter had been with me when Dr Singh had sketched these interrelationships (see chapters 11 & 18), so he was already on my wavelength. He then made a very practical suggestion:

"Why don't you use a Venn Diagram to illustrate the suppression of the immune system?"

Quickly I drew 3 circles and where they all overlapped in the centre I wrote "The patient's life circumstances". Then I encircled the entire diagram and labelled this outer circle the "circulatory system"; basically the bloodstream driven by our hearts.

Peter agreed, saying my sketch was simple and clear. After all it was the circulatory system that as he said,

"enabled good and bad stuff to get around the body."

Now what I had to figure out was where to place an overlay representing the gut. Dr Singh had told me that about 70% of the immune system is housed in the gut, so I decided that a significant brown shadow would illustrate the point I wanted to make (see Figure 7).

Prolonged undue tension and immune suppression

Having illustrated why my immune system had been weakened, I felt I needed to take my understanding of what might have occurred in May 2011 (see chapter 7) a step further. What I felt was critically important was to emphasise the part my dysfunctional gut had played in suppressing my immune system. After talking it over with Peter I decided a flow diagram would be the answer. I wanted to depict the series of events that had occurred, beginning with my mind's reaction to undue and prolonged tension. As Dr Singh had said *'it'* had occurred twice in my life; first in the Notre Dame library and again in 2010/2011 (see chapters 4 & 13).

My problem was that whenever I became tense my gut shut down. In my case it had become an involuntary reflex or response to the absence of readily available toilets. This bad gut habit is likely to have originated at the age of 5 when I started school. To this day I can clearly recall gagging in the primary school toilet block as the unbelievable stench from unflushed toilets engulfed me. Those toilets had to be avoided at all costs. This led to lifelong, severe constipation that I came to regard as par for the course. I thought the few sparse pellets I produced were normal. Eventually in later life I developed faecal impaction in my sigmoid colon and rectum. This caused damage in the form of pouches (see chapter 13). I'd also learnt from Dr Singh that partially undigested food could get lodged in these diverticula (pouches) which could lead to an increase in the growth of unhealthy microorganisms.

Given the pain and discomfort I felt in my right leg that May, I'm now in no doubt that I experienced a serious infection and associated inflammation. I also think, as does Dr Singh, that my unhealthy and damaged gut was the source of this infection. It was serendipitous that thanks to my persistence I received a course of macrodantin, an antibiotic (see chapter 2). This treatment instantly stopped the acute pain and throbbing, but I was left with stiff tendons, inflamed muscles and pinched nerves. The result was a weak, gammy right leg. Instead of accepting that an arthritis attack had had a permanent crippling affect, I resolved to fully restore my leg. This I achieved thanks to the skills of an exceptional physiotherapist (see chapter 10).

Now I felt I needed to construct a step-by-step diagram to depict this series of events, starting with my mind's reaction to prolonged stress and tension. Thanks to Dr Singh's sketches explaining the impact of stress on the body I was able to create a flowchart that depicted this chain of responses which had occurred twice in my life (see Figure 8).

In 1997 chronic constipation had caused throbbing wrists, painful feet which made me hobble, and "stickiness" between the upper vertebrae in my spine. Doctors had wondered whether I was developing *RA; Ankylosing Spondylitis* was even a possibility.

The toxic condition that developed in 2011 also had a widespread impact. X-rays revealed damaged joints in my right leg: a large cyst in my inner hip socket and minor cartilage damage in my knee. Added to this was my liver's initial, adverse reaction to a strong antifungal medication. Surprisingly once voriconazole was resumed my liver responded positively. The treatment ended up being very beneficial (see chapter 19).

Once my flowchart depicting a suppressed immune system was complete it outlined a 7-step process which included my weakened immune system becoming overloaded. There's no doubt in my mind that in *May 2011 a surge of toxins from my gut entered my bloodstream and briefly circulated.* My immune system did its best to respond and probably eventually got the better of a variety of nasty microorganisms thanks to macrodantin (an antibiotic) and voriconazole (an antifungal). However, it's apparent to me that irreparable damage had been done to my hip joint and surprise, surprise ... maybe even to my thyroid.

An infective agent: a possible underlying cause

My ever-inquisitive mind continued to ponder about My Concept and which bugs might have caused my issues. Had Dr Golledge, an expert in infectious disease, hoped to identify a microbial agent that was the culprit? After all, I recalled Dr Witherow saying it was possible for an infection to move from the bowel to the hip. It had also been suggested that a rotten tooth could result in an infection elsewhere in the body.

At bedtime one evening when Peter headed upstairs to our bedroom "eyrie" overlooking the treed gardens of UWA, I decided to continue my investigations. I recalled the dinner we'd enjoyed with Jim and Irene back in November (see chapter 16). Irene was well informed and had told me about the different types of prostheses used in hip replacements. We'd discussed the disastrous side-effects that had occurred with cobalt implants. Filaments from the cobalt joints had landed up deafening people as they got into their eardrums. Worse still, some people had developed dementia as some fine metal fragments had lodged in their brains.

Over our morning coffee I reminded Peter of those ghastly findings. To which he responded with some emotion.

"Good God ... stuff gets around in the body, doesn't it!"

"Yes, but that's not all. Jim also told us how a friend's joints had been damaged by fungus."

My mind had turned to Dr Crook's book about *"The yeast connection"* and the role *candida albicans* played. So I added,

"Maybe a fungus has damaged the cartilage in my hip joint?"

Ever practical, Peter simply said:

"Why don't you just ask Dr Singh?"

So, when I next saw him that April I asked:

"Do you think a bug of some sort, say a fungus, could have escaped from my bowel and damaged my hip? Maybe it has also affected my knee; even my liver?"

My GP patiently reminded me that a pathogen like a fungus can escape into the body, but our immune system usually kept a lid on it.

He then went on to add that,

"Fungal infections aren't very common. Mixed infections can also occur. It could've been bacteria."

"Well, could bacteria and/or a virus have buzzed around my body and affected other organs like my liver and thyroid?"

To this he simply shrugged and said, "You mean in the bloodstream."

"Yes, I've read that a virus like chicken pox remains lurking in our bodies. I know it latches onto our nerves and can re-emerge as shingles."

I was hoping he'd further elaborate, as I was wondering whether a microbial agent had indeed infected the synovial fluid in my right hip. Maybe that was why I'd received advice from the other side of the world (see chapter 2) stating:

"You have a cyst in your inner hip socket. You need to be referred to an orthopaedic surgeon to have a sample of synovial fluid collected from your joint."

True to his philosophy of "empowering the patient through the use of an educational approach", Dr Singh then recommended I add another book to my little collection of medical texts. It was a text written by microbiologists.

- Richardson, M.D. and Warnock, D.W., 2012: *Fungal Infection; diagnosis and management,* Wiley-Blackwell Publishers, Oxford, UK.

Previously he'd emphasised that there were trillions of microorganisms in the gut. Bacteria, viruses and fungi could all be possibilities, however, he drew my attention to my body's response to voriconazole. It was an antifungal which is different from an antibiotic and he felt the text on fungi would help me gain further understanding of my complex condition.

Conclusion

On my return home Peter was interested to know if Dr Singh had been able to further enlighten me regarding my complex condition. When I mentioned the medical text my GP had recommended he unhesitatingly encouraged me to buy it, rather than wait to borrow my GP's copy.

Peter understood my thinking about My Concept to that point. By synthesising what I'd experienced, together with graphs of telling changes in thyroid and liver function, I'd clarified my theory of what might've occurred. My idea of My Concept was crystallised in my flowchart depicting my suppressed immune system that couldn't control *a surge of toxins from my damaged gut* (see Figure 8).

For me this culminated in a harmful event that gave rise to inflammation, infection, ailments and a disease such as septic arthritis.

While I waited impatiently for the *Fungal infection text* to arrive, I again leafed through Dr Jenner's book which covered a range of different types of arthritis. The two that interested me were:

- Septic arthritis
- Fungal arthritis

I noted that with fungal arthritis sometimes only one joint is affected. My intuition told me this could be me and my right hip. I wasn't suffering from a disease that affected multiple joints. Amongst the fungi most often responsible, candida was listed.

Chapter 21 CANDIDA ALBICANS (May 2013)

Analysis of blood test results for Liver and Thyroid function had helped me consolidate my understanding of My Concept in the form of a flowchart (see Figure 8). My idea was that a surge of toxins of some sort had seeped into my bloodstream and overwhelmed my weakened immune system. This gave rise to inflammation and/or infection. What hadn't been determined was whether a finger could be pointed at the chief culprits.

If I'd simply focussed on a possible mixed infection that had done a huge amount of damage to the cartilage in my right hip socket, the ramifications of my complex condition would've been overlooked. By the end of 2012 I'd started to realise that the infection wasn't restricted to just my hip. It was likely to have been far more widespread. An agent of some sort could have been carried in my bloodstream to tissues and organs at quite a distance from my sigmoid colon and rectum. My Concept was the cornerstone of my complex condition which had probably given rise to serious consequences.

Benign transient candidemia

The *Fungal infection* text Dr Singh had recommended arrived within a week. Immediately I began reading and soon became utterly absorbed. All my 2011 ailments (see chapter 19) were described. To find my complex condition clearly outlined in an authoritative medical text brought a huge sense of relief. Finally I hoped I would be able to identify a key infective culprit.

By the end of that day the text *"Fungal Infection"* was bristling with post-it tabs marking relevant pages heavily highlighted in yellow. Page after page had resonated with me, what I'd experienced and my understanding of *'it'*. I felt that my theory wasn't fantastical after all as there was a possible medical explanation for the symptoms I'd experienced.

The section I'd immediately turned to was entitled *Candidosis;* apparently this condition is also referred to as *Candidiasis.* I was able to recognise it thanks to the 1986 text written by Dr Crook (see chapter 6). But it was clear to see why Dr Singh had wanted me to obtain a more recent medical text where discussion of the topic was based on clinical data. Over the past 30 years advances had been made in the diagnosis and treatment of fungal infections.

I discovered that much like pain can be divided into two categories (acute and chronic), so could this fungal condition be either short lived and transient or it could persist long-term. Richardson and Warnock's book went on to state that previously a condition called "transient candidemia" had been considered benign, requiring no treatment. However, this approach was now considered hazardous as they'd uncovered a "high incidence of metastatic complications" following the spread of *Candida* species through the bloodstream. Of these fungal species *Candida albicans* was named as the leading cause of *Candida* bloodstream infection, or to use medical jargon "*Candida albicans* is the principal aetological agent".

It began to dawn on me that the reason I'd received excellent medical attention throughout 2012 was because three astute doctors had felt my case was more serious than I realised. The doctor who initially sounded an alarm was Dr Brennan (see chapter 5). Not only had he encouraged me to contact Dr Singh, but he'd emphasised,

"You must come back in two years. This is very bad."

When I'd first met Dr Golledge in mid-2011 I'd also noticed that he'd not been totally relaxed. As I'd left his surgery he'd thrust his card at me saying,

"Come back and see me. Here, take my card."

Disseminated candidosis (Systemic candidiasis)

When I'd peppered Dr Singh with questions as to the possibility of a fungus buzzing around the body, he'd mentioned the bloodstream. Now in the *Fungal infection* text I'd read that bloodstream infections can be caused by *Candida albicans.* Such infections occur when yeasts (one celled microbes) belonging to the *genus Candida* become widespread. These yeasts can be seeded in organs such as the liver, spleen and kidneys. My liver tests had strongly indicated there was hepatic involvement. Maybe yeasts had also "got my thyroid" as I'd heard Dr Golledge mutter.

At last I realised why I'd been given a blood test for *Systemic Candidiasis*, but the mystery was that the results were negative. This finding wouldn't have surprised a highly experienced, clinical microbiologist. The term transient was warranted because these one-celled yeasts didn't stay in the bloodstream for very long, which made the condition difficult to diagnose [my emphasis]. Instead the authors of the *Fungal infection* text stated that "the decision to begin antifungal treatment should be based on clinical signs and risk factors, as blood cultures are usually negative." Truly it was fortunate that I'd done my homework and compiled a personal list of my symptoms and risk factors. For me the most significant of these factors was a damaged bowel (see chapter 12).

A statement in the text confirmed that "cases arise from the translocation of organisms across the wall of the intestinal tract. Haematogenous spread [bloodstream dissemination] can then lead to tissue invasion where the single cell yeast forms [of *Candida*] become imbedded in organs."

The following two statements made me really take notice:

- "Cutaneous [skin] lesions are useful clinical signs of acute disseminated candidosis."
- "Late complications include septic arthritis."

No wonder my tale of ailments in early 2011 had begun with skin issues: spots, rashes, scaling, cracks and puckering. I could also remember that certain movements involving my right hip had made me feel a bit nauseous (see chapter 5).

The AIDs epidemic and advances in medical knowledge

Reading about candidosis in an authoratitive medical text had brought me peace of mind as an explanation for what I felt occurred in 2011/2012 had been provided. Yet this explanation wasn't new, as Dr Crook had already described such a condition in 1983 when the first edition of *The yeast connection* had been published. Unfortunately his work was largely based on clinical observation, so it was not widely accepted by the medical establishment.

I began to wonder what had provided the impetus for the collection of clinical data by microbiologists such as Richardson and Warnock. The answer was the AIDS epidemic which took off in the western world in the early 1980s.

If I was to do everything within my power to maintain my health and keep this yeast pestilence at bay, I had to know what I was up against. Maybe I needed to find out more about the AIDS epidemic. What had this deadly disease got to do with fungal infections? Again it was Peter who came up with a helpful suggestion.

"Have you heard of a film called: *And the band played on*? It's received rave reviews and covers the outbreak of AIDS in San Francisco."

With that, our evening entertainment was decided. I found the film enthralling, but also disturbing. The impact of the disease as it swept through the gay community was frightful. What disturbed me were the challenges that faced a young doctor desperate to do all within his power to alleviate the suffering. Once virile young men had rapidly succumbed to infections and available treatments were limited.

The film was based on an award winning bestseller by a journalist:

- Shilts, R., 1988: *And the band played on,* St. Martin's Griffin, New York, USA.

This well researched and detailed account was soon added to my library and before long it was also bristling with post-it notes. Randy Shilts was an impressive writer; a past master at using evocative expression. In a few sentences he graphically reinforced the importance of a strong immune system:

"When modern medicine learned how to intentionally suppress the immune system [my emphasis] so the body would not reject transplanted kidneys and hearts, *Pneumocystis* flared sporadically, eager to take advantage of any opportunity to thrive in its preferred ecological niche, the lung. The disease, however, would disappear spontaneously once the immune system was restored. And the little creature would then lurk on the fringes, lying dormant until opportunity allowed it to burst forth and follow the biological dictate to grow and multiply."

Pneumonia wasn't the only symptom these ill men presented with. Many were also suffering from "a wicked case of candidiasis". Randy Shilts didn't pull any punches. His graphic descriptions of candidiasis in the dying were horrific.

What Mathew Modine (the actor portraying the young doctor's plight) didn't have to hand were a suite of azole drugs. So it was my good fortune that by 2011 the pharmacy up the road, within the Charlie Gairdner hospital complex was well stocked with voriconazole (Vfend).

Problematic diagnosis

It appeared that liver invasion with candida species was almost impossible to diagnose prior to treatment. According to Richardson and Warnock nothing may be discernible on radiographic images and liver function abnormalities may be mild or absent. Most patients are asymptomatic.

Nevertheless, it made me ever so slightly alarmed to think Dr Golledge had spotted symptoms that warranted such a strong anti-fungal. His diagnostic treatment must have confirmed his shrewd assessment. After all, a serious hepatic (liver) reaction had occurred, in spite of liver function tests indicating nothing untoward. As Richardson and Warnock state, this pointed to "deep-organ candidosis"; a "critical diagnostic sign of acute disseminated candidosis." They go on to elaborate, saying that single cell yeast forms can spread through the bloodstream and invade tissues. Apparently, these microscopic yeast spores could become embedded in organs such as the liver (see Figure 9).

You'd think this information would've satisfied me. But no, I then decided to search the web to discover what hepatic candidiasis looked like. An academic paper in a radiology journal gave me more images than Peter could stomach looking at. Photos of thin sections from a liver showed white patches; microabscesses filled with yeast forms.

Surely my case wasn't anything like what was depicted in the radiology journal? But actually it might have been. Some cases are only confirmed after life has ended; at the time of autopsy.

The academic paper went on to support Dr Golledge's treatment, stating that "the inflammatory response was pivotal in defining organ involvement." How fortunate I was to have received "prophylactic antifungal therapy" with Vfend; a relatively new antifungal that was the best available.

When Dr Golledge stopped his voriconazole treatment towards the end of 2012 I'd felt slightly unnerved, particularly as the beneficial effect on my thyroid was short term. Just as he predicted I did eventually develop hypothyroidism, but fortunately it's easily treated. What delighted me though was the way my liver function had been improved.

At the start of 2013 the only issue that remained was my right hip. Even though I'd resumed brisk, pain-free, long walks my doctors remained pessimistic, as further cartilage destruction was likely; probably inevitable. It became apparent that efforts to restore severely damaged cartilage would be futile; my time and energy would be better spent on prevention of damage to other joints. To do this I needed to come to grips with the possible mechanisms that had resulted in an exceedingly painful infection.

Intestinal candidosis, gut permeability and bloodstream dissemination

Towards the end of 2011 I'd drawn up my own list of personal risk factors (see chapter 12) which had impressed my GP. It surprised me that Richardson and Warnock only briefly and pessimistically mentioned possible risks relating to invasive candidosis, stating

"Many risk factors have been identified, but few of these factors are preventable or modifiable."

Undeterred I began to revise my list of factors in light of what I'd learnt from their *Fungal infection* text. To clarify *My Concept* of what might have occurred I decided to link my risks to the mechanisms involved in the dispersal of noxious, microbial critters like *C.albicans* through the bloodstream to remote organs and of course to joints.

1. **GI tract candidosis:** Excessive colonisation (overgrowth) of *C.albicans* in the large bowel. Possible causes: broad spectrum antibiotics, unhealthy modern diet, food source (organic waste) in pockets (diverticula), beneficial bacteria outnumbered.

2. **GI perforation:** Microscopic tears in weak abnormal pouches of gut due to excessive pressure resulting from faecal impaction.
3. **Immune system briefly overwhelmed:** An uncontrolled number of hostile microbes cross the epithelial barrier and enter circulation. Microscopic one-celled spores like *C. albicans* travel in yeast form through the bloodstream via portal venous circulation (believed to be a common route).
4. **Tissue invasion:** *C. albicans* is polymorphic and pathogenic; i.e. its growth form changes (see Figure 9) and it produces true hyphae once it's embedded in tissues, organs and possibly my inner hip socket.

It's my belief that the 4 steps I've outlined above could provide a possible explanation for an endogenous infection in my right leg; i.e. the culprits were noxious microbes that escaped from weak points on the right side of my large bowel.

The question I then asked myself was which risk factor was the primary cause. What had predisposed me to developing an infection? To my mind the answer is obvious. My dysfunctional gut was the underlying cause of my problems. Given that 70% of the immune system is located in the gut, I felt that a suppressed immune response was part and parcel of the "infective problems" I encountered in 2011/2012. My theory &/or explanation is that my clogged gut had hamstrung my immune response. My enfeebled immune system couldn't adequately defend me; my resistance to infection was weak.

Before Dr Golledge and Dr Singh took me under their wing in the second half of 2011 I was tense, anxious and frightened. I'd suffered extremely intense pain which was thankfully short-lived. My mind was filled with the following questions:

- What had caused the extremely intense pain?
- Why was it acute (short-lived)?
- Would these attacks be "ongoing" as I'd been told?
- Would it affect other joints?

- Could the underlying cause be identified and treated?
- Could this *arthritis* be stopped?

Instinctively by 2013 I knew, as Dr Golledge had reassured me, that I was doing the right thing. However, maybe I would have to wait 10 years before I could confidently claim that as Dr Jenner predicted, I'd "driven my arthritis into complete remission."

Chapter 22 "A GREY AREA OF MEDICINE" (Jun 2013)

Having absorbed all that Richardson and Warnock had to say in their *Fungal infection* text about the *C. albicans* pestilence, I came to the realisation that this fungus was not to be trifled with. It was polymorphic and had the sinister ability to alter its form to suit the circumstances. This microbe was also opportunistic and if there was a microscopic tear in the bowel wall it could slip into the bloodstream in the form of a single celled microscopic yeast, and travel throughout the body. Upon reaching a destination it could morph into a hypha and embed itself in an organ such as the liver(see Figure 9).

I couldn't have achieved this understanding without the Thesaurus online, as the text was filled with medical terms that a lay person wouldn't be familiar with. However, it gave me a great sense of satisfaction to be able to express *My Concept* using doctors' jargon; viz.

A transient candidemia episode had occurred in May 2011 which was not benign as my immune system was weak. The chief aetiological agent was Candida albicans; a normally harmless commensal that resides in our GI tract. Microscopic perforations in my colon (damaged by faecal impaction) had enabled this polymorphic, pathogenic fungus to opportunistically translocate across the epithelial wall of my sigmoid colon and rectum (see Figure 13). Subsequent haematogenous dissemination had led to tissue invasion. Single celled yeast spores had adhered to distant mucosal surfaces and become embedded in an organ like my liver by morphing into hyphae.

Basically what I'd eventually clarified for myself was that my arthritic hip was the result of an endogenous infection (an internal source; viz. my gut), so the causative agents could have been mixed – fungi, bacteria or viruses. What was sobering was the realisation that the infection hadn't been limited to just my hip. This made me recall another recurrent manifestation of *C. albicans* that I'd experienced for decades, but that'd got particularly bad in 2010. It was thrush, a superficial form of candidiasis, that frequently occurs in the female genital tract. It occurred to me that the unpleasant yeasty condition which had plagued me for years, had simply vanished. I suspected it was thanks to the miraculous treatment I'd received in 2011 and 2012.

A GP trained in Traditional Chinese Medicine & Modern Western Medicine

At the start of my health journey early in 2011 the GPs I'd sought help from had initially dismissed my health issues as trivial. A dermatologist had even apologised saying,

"I know it's frustrating when people can't help you."

This had resulted in my stumbling from pillar to post until fortuitously in the middle of the year I'd met a functional medicine doctor. This GP had instantly gone into action with tests, printed information, provision of supplements (notably a large daily dose of vitamin D), and advice on a nutritious high fibre diet to remedy my dysfunctional gut (see chapter 8). His recommendations and treatments were very much in line with what I'd learnt from Dr Campbell and Dr Crook's books. When he'd told me he'd had *'it'* and he could stabilise *'it'*, I'd been left nonplussed. However, thankfully he was absolutely right as he helped me turn a corner and started me on a road towards what I feel was a miraculous recovery. Why then was this effective treatment not widely available?

As my biennial pap test was due I decided to make the most of an opportunity to hopefully obtain more information about what the endocrinologist had termed a "complex condition." At least Professor Walsh had been prepared to describe my health issue, rather than cryptically referring to *'it'* (see chapter 15).

By 2013 I'd learnt to make optimal use of my allotted appointment times with doctors and specialists. So before picking up the phone I compiled a list of the questions that were at the forefront of my mind. Given the *Fungal infection* text had provided me with current clinical information about candidiasis, my questions didn't focus on the disease as such, but rather on why it had been such a struggle to find doctors who could help me. My list turned out to be quite long, so I landed up booking a double appointment at a large clinic in a neighbouring suburb. The clinic had lady GPs, but more importantly it was a medical practice that covered both Chinese Medicine and Western Medicine.

Together with my questionnaire I added my risk factors and my summary of what I now referred to as My Concept. As I headed off to the large clinic I half thought that the new doctor I was to meet might find all the material rather confronting. But thankfully this was not the case. The wonderfully pleasant GP turned out to be forthcoming and exceedingly helpful as I launched into my quest for more answers.

- *The last 18 months have been eventful, but also confusing as I was perplexed by doctors' responses. I found the lack of clarity unnerving, so I landed up putting together these risk factors and developed my own theory/concept.*

"For a non-medical person it's remarkable what information you've managed to piece together, and what you've achieved."

Her compliment was like balm for the soul. It boosted my self-esteem, which at times had received a bit of a battering, especially in early 2011.

- *Why did I struggle to find someone who could help? When I eventually met the functional medicine doctor he'd instantly known what measures were needed to correct my condition. He seemed to know without even asking, that I had a serious gut health issue.*

"Your medical history would've indicated what the problem was. I can see that thrush has been an ongoing nuisance for many years. Is it still troubling you?"

- *No, amazingly it's vanished. I've almost forgotten I ever had it!*

"This shows your positive response to treatment has confirmed the candidiasis diagnosis."

- *This is the first time my complex condition's been given a name. Why did so many doctors just persist with a perplexing reference to 'it'?*

"Well *'it'* is not officially recognised by modern medicine as there's limited scientific evidence. Actually it's a grey area of Western Medicine and is regarded as harmless. Most of the time it simply passes. Usually only very sick people with compromised immune systems receive treatment."

- *Why then did Dr Golledge put me on voriconazole?*

"Maybe your condition was for a long time subclinical, but you must've reached a tipping point. Dr Golledge probably recognised that *C. albicans* was getting the upperhand and your immune system was losing control. You needed his voriconazole to push it back. Now they hope your immune system will hold it; i.e. keep it at bay. You're very lucky to have found the right doctors to help you as your condition isn't recognised by most doctors."

- *Is this why my pharmacist recommended a Chinese doctor to me who'd also received modern medical training? He referred to him as a "cross-over" doctor. Is it possible that Traditional Chinese medicine is better than modern Western Medicine?*

"No, modern medicine is very well equipped to deal with major life- threatening conditions. Your condition is unpleasant, but it's not life-threatening. However, Traditional Chinese medicine is better at providing preventative (prophylactic) treatment for some chronic conditions."

- *Well, Dr Golledge told me I was well which meant I was doing something right, but I don't know for sure what that is. Am I deluding myself to think I can heal myself and repair my hip?*

"Yes and no. You can definitely prevent future candidiasis outbreaks by sticking to the hunter-gatherer, low-sugar diet that Dr Singh recommended (see chapter 14). But it's doubtful that you'll be able to repair your severely damaged hip cartilage with Joint-Food. Research shows only a slight improvement in 30% of both humans and animals. Fractures mend, but not cartilage."

By that stage time had run out. I would have to return for the pap smear. As I left this wonderful doctor gave me one last piece of advice, saying there was a well-known Chinese proverb: "No illness – short life. One illness – long life."

You mean if I learn from past bad eating habits and maintain a healthy low-sugar diet, I can look forward to a long life?

To this she simply smiled and nodded. She'd given me an understanding and some peace of mind. But I still wondered if there was anything else I could do to help my immune system keep candidiasis at bay.

Chapter 23 ASSOCIATED AILMENTS (Jul 2013)

By mid-2013 I'd learnt a lot about my complex condition by questioning GPs and specialists, and of course by reading. The clinical observations outlined in depth by Dr Crook in *The yeast connection* had been largely validated by the hospital data Richardson and Warnock had collated. Nevertheless, the lady GP had made me very aware that I mustn't assume modern medicine knew everything. There were a lot of "unknowns", however even if exact mechanisms weren't fully understood many links or associations between conditions were recognised. A number of such conditions or minor ailments had preceded the onset of my excruciating arthritis attacks.

Thrush (candidiasis)

Thanks to my appointment for a biennial pap test I'd been reminded that thrush which had plagued me for decades had simply vanished. I'd probably always had *C. albicans* present in both my genital and GI tracts, but as Richardson and Warnock explained this normal colonisation within our body could grow out of control. Factors like stress and some medications (e.g. broad spectrum antibiotics &/or corticosteroids) may disturb the balance between good and bad microbes. A small presence of *C. albicans* was acceptable, but it shouldn't be allowed to overrun and turn into an infestation.

Dermatitis

Another issue which had prompted me to seek medical attention in early 2011 had been a type of dermatitis. This complaint would also have been forgotten if it wasn't for an entry I'd made in my journal. I'd simply jotted down: "Picking skin off my face with tweezers."

Odd changes to my skin had started to bother me. Severe dandruff too was no longer just a bit of a nuisance. Then there were the peculiar eczema-like patches that had appeared behind my right knee and near my right hip.

At around that time I could also no longer ignore my sore hip. Thankfully a perceptive dermatologist put two and two together. He was well informed and knew of the links between what he said was "a yeast infection" and associated conditions; viz. dermatitis, dandruff, eczema/psoriasis, thyroiditis and arthritis. At the end of my appointment with him I'd been given a request for a blood test to check thyroid function and a referral to see Professor John Walsh, the endocrinologist (see chapter 15).

Costochondritis

Of all the weird and wonderful ailments that manifested themselves, by far the most frightening was costochondritis. Towards the middle of 2012 my voriconazole treatment was again well underway, but at a very low dose of 50mg in the morning and again later in the evening. My body had responded so well that I truly felt cured of absolutely everything; even arthritic symptoms in my right leg had pretty much disappeared.

As I felt fit and well I enthusiastically accepted Peter's offer of a trip to Melbourne with him. It would be an opportunity to catch up with my sister after all. The business meetings Peter had to attend were on a Monday, so by flying over to the east coast on the Friday we'd give ourselves the weekend to visit the many tourist attractions Melbourne had to offer.

Before heading off the next morning to explore museums, art galleries and markets we first scouted for a good pair of walking shoes for me. In a city like Melbourne this was an absolute pleasure; there were so many shoe-stores we had trouble deciding where to start. Once my feet were well equipped to go pounding, we set off. It was so enjoyable we didn't notice time passing, or the distance covered. By the end of the day we estimated we'd covered 5.5 kilometres. With great satisfaction I made an entry in my new "Walking Records" which had displaced my old "Pain Records" from 2011.

All the exercise meant I looked forward to an early night and a good, sound sleep. But it was not to be. In the wee hours of the morning, just before sunrise a strong, aching pain in the centre of my chest woke me. With immense consternation Peter leapt up and brought me a glass of water and a couple of aspirins. The discomfort was so severe I had trouble pulling myself up against the pillows to take a sip.

Of course both of us immediately thought "heart attack", but fortunately that wasn't the case. Surprisingly the painkillers brought swift relief and after a leisurely room-service breakfast I was back to my cheerful self and good to go. We planned to meet my sister Susan and her husband Martin in the botanical gardens for lunch.

The rest of our Melbourne trip passed without a hitch and by the end of the week I was back home and catching up with a backlog of laundry. As Peter hadn't returned with me I had the weekend to myself which I didn't mind at all. He'd flown on from Sydney to South America and I was used to such extended business trips. They were simply a part of being married to a man in the mining game.

That weekend though I could've done with his support. As I happily daydreamed while hanging washing in the cool afternoon seabreeze I was jolted by another sharp, painful shock. In an instant I became stranded; immobile under the washing line as another severe attack gripped me. I gasped as I felt a tightness that made it difficult for me to breath. All I could do was remain quietly in the shade of the pear tree listening to the rustling leaves.

Eventually the pain eased, but I was left feeling alarmed and anxious. Should I call someone? Peter would've been well over the Pacific by then. There was my son, but I thought he'd mentioned an AFL match at the Subiaco stadium, just a short stroll from where he lived.

What if I had suffered a heart attack? Time would be of the essence, so I decided there and then to head straight up to emergency at my nearby Charlie Gairdner Hospital. Within a matter of minutes I was being attended to by a fine young man who told me he'd just returned from a conference at the Groote Schuur Hospital in Cape Town. No doubt he recognised my South African accent which I haven't managed to lose despite the fact that since 1980 Australia has been well and truly my home.

It didn't take long before he relaxed and talked things through with me. I think the voriconazole medication I was on had helped him reach an assessment of my troubling complaint which he named costochondritis. He said the pain from this inflammatory condition was very similar to that of a heart attack. However, this pain wasn't at all serious as it didn't lead to any permanent damage. Unhappily it probably would recur from time to time and when it did I should simply take ibuprofen. Naturally I wondered what had caused it, but unfortunately it fell into medicine's idiopathic category. It was another obscure, grey area. Even though he felt confident about his diagnosis, this calm and friendly doctor told me he'd send me for an ECG just to make sure I was okay, before letting me return home. And then last but not least he added:

"When you see your GP for a follow up you should ask him to check your vitamin D levels. Costochondritis has been linked to RA and Ank. Spond."

Fibromyalgia

Many years had passed since I'd experienced a brush with what might have been rheumatoid arthritis &/or ankylosing spondylitis (see chapter 4). When we'd lived in Kalgoorlie I'd experienced discomfort towards the top of my spine which had also rendered me momentarily immobile. I recalled asking Peter to massage the area between my shoulder blades. Again the discomfort had passed and almost been completely forgotten. On this occasion though I decided not to simply ignore what had occurred.

With time alone that weekend I returned to leafing through the books in my study; to shelves burgeoning with texts on arthritis. I came across a description of fibromyalgia which matched what I'd experienced in Kalgoorlie. Interestingly it too was an elusive inflammatory condition that at one stage doctors thought wasn't even real.

Transient Candidemia

I found myself being drawn back to the books on yeasts and fungi. Crook described symptoms that he connected to candidiasis saying "patients might experience pain or tightness in their chests." In the *Fungal infection* text it was stated that,

"Costochondral involvement can be a frequent and characteristic finding."

This got me thinking that perhaps repeated acute, pervasive candidemia episodes had caused inflammation not just in my thyroid and liver (see chapter 19), but also in the cartilage that connected my ribs to my breastbone. Just like with Alice in Wonderland this extraordinarily complex condition of mine simply became "curiouser and curiouser."

I found it simply fascinating and couldn't help but continue my investigations. When I read that inflammation is a frequent and characteristic finding related to candidosis, I made up my mind to take action; to continue to steer my own course.

In 2012 voriconazole was the best treatment available to treat candidosis. With this knowledge it made sense for me to contact Dr Golledge. I still had his card which I'd not used up until then, but I remembered how he'd urged me to take it. I hoped my simple text message wouldn't be too much of an intrusion. Briefly I outlined the painful and frightening costochondritis attacks which I'd been told would recur. To date the Vfend treatment had been extraordinarily beneficial, but my current dose was very low. Would he agree to my increasing it slightly?

In an instant I received a response and it was positive. "Your liver is recovering well so I'm comfortable with your increasing the dose to 100mg in the morning and 100mg in the evening. But you must get your liver tested again in two weeks' time. Make an appointment with Dr Singh and I will see you again in July."

That evening I didn't have to go through the tedious process of sawing the large white Vfend tablet in half now that the dose had doubled. Instead I confidently swallowed the hard tablet whole as instinctively I knew Dr Golledge's treatment would do the trick. As it turned out my blood test results revealed just that. A marked downward step change had occurred in response to the increased voriconazole dose (see Figure 6). My liver improved and so did the inflammation around my breastbone. To this day those frightful costochondritis attacks have not returned.

Hepatitis and Thyroiditis

My complex condition that appeared to be associated with candidosis, eventually involved six separate locations in my body where inflammation occurred; viz. fibromyalgia between my shoulder blades, inflamed breastbone cartilage, an hepatic liver, looming thyroiditis, and an inflammation/infection in two joints (right hip and knee). Thankfully the 2012 voriconazole treatment put a stop to all the pain and discomfort associated with this inflammatory condition. It even improved my liver function, but damage to my thyroid and hip cartilage eventually could not be reversed.

At my next appointment with Dr Singh he'd received the pleasing results from my blood tests. Sadly though he was dubious about the chances of my hip cartilage repairing itself. He also told me that thyroid antibodies tended to go up and down. Sometimes the condition spontaneously improved, but that wasn't very common. However he did provide me with a natural therapy called thyroplex which would help my sluggish thyroid in the short term.

Of course I also let him know about my heart adventure and the ECG I'd had. With that he briefly referred to my records and reassured me that all was well, just as the young doctor from Charlie Gairdner had predicted. This led on to the topic of vitamin D, a supplement that Dr Golledge had also suggested. Recent research was showing that this vitamin helped the body resist infections.

Just the previous year I'd received gut treatment from a functional medicine doctor who'd immediately placed me on a high 5,000 IU daily dose of vitamin D3 (see chapter 8). As the voriconazole treatment had been so effective Dr Singh felt such a high dose was no longer necessary. Instead he recommended dropping back to 1,000 IUs as I also took ostelin+VitD3 to help stave off osteoporosis. Then I remembered Campbell's cod liver oil, a recommendation dating back to 1997 (see chapter 4). This traditional medication has been used for centuries as a preventative measure against vitamin D deficiency.

Surely from all these links with conditions possibly related to a transient form of candidosis, it would be reasonable for me to infer that my hip issue was indeed "an infective problem".

Septic Arthritis

Of all my conditions that appeared in 2011, it was septic arthritis that had galvanised me into taking determined action. In addition to all the information I'd found in Dr Jenner's book, I also started sourcing information from material published on the internet by the University of Maryland Medical School. It intrigued me to find the following statement:

"Septic arthritis is inflammation of a joint due to bacterial, or fungal (such as *Candida albicans*) infection. Disease causing microorganisms spread through the bloodstream to a joint. The most common sites for this type of infection are the knee and the hip."

I went on to discover from the Johns Hopkins University website that,

"Septic arthritis can [also] develop when an infection, such as a urinary tract infection, spreads through the bloodstream to a joint."

For me all this information hung together logically and provided a clear explanation for the excruciating attacks in early 2011. Doctors weren't to blame for struggling to come up with an immediate diagnosis as I was guilty of not revealing my unpleasant brown urine and black stools. Eventually the treatment I received covered all possibilities as viruses, mycobacteria and fungi could all have been causative agents.

Conclusion

As Dr Golledge had said: "I was an important sample of one." I think that from all my accumulated evidence it could be suggested that Dr Crook was right:

"My health problems were yeast-connected."

My theory/concept is that a transient candidemia episode which I experienced in May 2011 had been pervasive. To my mind a logical explanation for my symptoms was that chronic mucosal candidiasis (definitely in my genital tract; possibly in my GI tract) became invasive and had spread through my bloodstream. Inflammation had occurred in my right leg (septic arthritis), in cartilage connecting my ribs to my sternum (costochondritis), in my liver (hepatitis) and my thyroid (thyroiditis). My thinking is that the areas of my body that had become inflamed were related to this candidemia episode (transient yeast infection) and were clearly not the result of suggested explanations such as trauma &/or "wear and tear". This understanding enabled me to focus my attention on means to boost my immune system to prevent a recurrence of a condition that wasn't life-threatening but had been very unpleasant and painful.

Chapter 24 PRIMARY PREVENTION (Jul – Dec 2013)

Back in May 2011 when Dr Brennan, the gastroenterologist, had alluded to the role of the immune system I was mystified as I'd been told my hip problem was due to the mechanical wearing away of the cartilage (see chapter 3). These conflicting explanations prompted me to seek a second opinion from another GP, and then I went on to obtain further opinions from specialists. None of these physicians ever gave me a definitive diagnosis. Instead I was told that the medical profession "didn't really know". However, they did appear to know what I should do to keep my unpleasant and painful condition at bay, as I was repeatedly given a single bit of definitive advice; viz. "keep supporting your immune system".

Well I'm sure this advice was given with the best of intentions, but I wasn't given much guidance as to what measures I should take. It was all a bit unnerving, but fortunately I could again turn to my knowledgeable GP. Hopefully he'd be able to further enlighten me. He'd fully approved of my personal list of risk factors so they would provide a starting point (see chapter 12). By the middle of 2013 I felt confident that I was achieving remission and the fact that I'd addressed those risk factors must have contributed to my progress. Of course the *Ank.Spond.* genetic marker was a factor I couldn't change, but the lifestyle factors could be addressed.

FACTORS THAT WEAKENED MY IMMUNE SYSTEM:

1.Gut Dysfunction

I decided that for me my dysfunctional gut was my primary risk factor. Back in 1997 by following Campbell's guidelines I'd achieved relief from arthritic symptoms almost immediately (see chapter 4). What tops his list is "alleviating constipation". In his book he describes arthritis as a "toxic condition" and to flush toxins from my system I needed to fix the chronic constipation. This advice is echoed by Phelps as she states in her book that "adequate elimination of toxins is vital." The treatment she advises is simply a high-fibre diet. However, for me such advice didn't suffice. My case was extreme. The constipation that I had lived with for more than 50 years was off the charts.

After almost a lifetime my mind had become capable of overruling what should have been an automatic gut function. Peristalsis in my large bowel basically ground to a halt. The involuntary wave-like contractions that should have pushed digested waste out of my body no longer worked. Even Campbell's recommendation of a daily tablespoon of cod liver oil didn't do the trick.

Eventually I'd had to resort to using laxatives to outwit the hold my mind had over my gut. If I was travelling, a couple of senna tablets taken in the morning would not produce any results. My gut simply remained shut down as it knew that I'd be out and about and clean, acceptable toilets might not be readily available. Instead I learnt to always carry the little senna tablets in my handbag, ready to be accessed when alerted by a reminder on my phone at 4pm. It was crucial that I took them on an empty stomach well before dinner. Peristalsis would then reliably kick into gear during the night as I slept; my mind simply couldn't interfere.

As Dr Singh had impressed on me that a daily bowel motion (BM) was essential I didn't give up on the idea of retraining my gut. But my GP wasn't in favour of laxatives. By pure chance one day in May 2012 I learnt from a magazine about coffee being used as a laxative. Before experimenting I double checked to see whether this was wise by looking at the Johns Hopkins medical website. I was delighted to discover that there are several reasons why coffee could be good for one. The Hopkins nutrition experts stated that coffee contains antioxidants which may reduce inflammation and protect against disease.

With this newfound knowledge I soon discovered that two strong mugs of coffee first thing in the morning worked a treat. Soon daily dumps became a matter of course ... they still are.

Evidently the hold my mind had over the bodily function of my gut needed to be relaxed. It seemed logical to establish the reasons why my gut was misbehaving. Following further research I came up with the following:

- *Address my gut's response to travel* (With my daily BM routine altered, elimination of waste ground to a halt. Fortunately strong morning coffee solved that problem.)
- *No access to a toilet when needed – forward planning was required.*
- *Overcome the dislike of using communal toilets* (I didn't like going in strange places and preferred the comfort of my own home.)
- *Ensure I was comfortably seated – clean public toilet seat if necessary.*

This was essential as I'd perfected the technique of suspending myself well above the offensive, strange seat. All very well if just a quick pee was needed. But a poo ... oh no ... not today ... maybe not tomorrow ... maybe next week?

(Note: Enders emphasises in her book that the western porcelain bowl doesn't facilitate an easy BM as squatting is the natural pooing position. She advises leaning forward to compensate; even to rock to and fro if necessary. Could we learn something from the Muslim tradition? Their toilet at UWA is made of porcelain, but it's a smallish opening in the floor.)

The manner in which my mind unconsciously suppressed the urge to poo isn't unheard of. One morning I learnt about a similar phenomenon when listening to the ABC health report. A clinical study had been carried out to investigate the impact of long flights on the health of pilots. The findings were extraordinary. Close to 200 pilots had had to be admitted to hospital, not to treat faecal impaction, but to deal with bladders filled to bursting point. They had to be catheterised to relieve the pressure.

Having dealt with my biggest hurdle, I turned my attention to seeing if I could do something about the damage faecal impaction had caused to the wall of my bowel.

2.Gut permeability

In May 2011 I first heard the word "diverticulosis" mentioned when Dr Singh's young colleague told me what my colonoscopy procedure had revealed. When I'd asked what it was he'd cheerily said that they were small sacks spotted in the wall of my right colon; apparently lots of people had them. It was only when I read up on diverticular disease in Phelp's tome that I learnt more and started to develop part of what would become my theory which I have referred to as My Concept.

Those small sacks or diverticula (pouches) had been caused by the hard, compacted bunches of stool in my sigmoid and rectum (see Figure 4). According to the Cleveland Clinic's website these abnormal pouches are weak and can "enable normal colonic bacteria to reach the peritoneal cavity; a very thin membrane which provides pathways for blood vessels". Could these weak sections have enabled infectious microbes to enter my bloodstream and escape to other parts of my body? I learnt that most of the time the presence of these hostile agents caused no harm, and Dr Singh had reassured me that they were repelled by a healthy immune response if they escaped into the body. But my brown urine and black stools indicated my immune system at the time was far from healthy and robust. Surely wouldn't this explain why my right leg had throbbed and disturbed my sleep?

Eager to restore my gut lining I started by finding out which parts of the body could repair themselves. Of course a cut in the skin can mend, even with barely a sign if stitched together by a surgeon. So what about the gut barrier? I'd heard it referred to as our body's inner skin. To me it seemed feasible that it too could heal itself, especially if I continued with my newfound habit of daily BMs. There'd be no more pressure; no more stretched distortions. In my mind's eye I envisaged those pouches given time, steadily shrinking and eventually shrivelling up; possibly even disappearing.

Later on I found out that my damaged bowel with its pouches had created an ideal habitat for noxious microbes to colonise. Undigested waste could easily have lodged in those pockets and provided rotting material to nourish those pesky critters. Early on in 2011 a GP had warned me that a colonoscopy wouldn't "clean me out". So what would? By chance I heard about turmeric and added it to my list of breakfast supplements. What happened at follow up loo times slightly repulsed me. Unwelcome guests in my gut that looked like mini jelly fish were expelled. What exactly they were I'll never know, but as the 2011 gut treatment continued, much to my relief their appearances became few and far between. Towards the end of 2011, once I'd begun Dr Golledge's voriconazole treatment I saw the shiny, glossy blobs for one last time. Then to my relief they were gone. Of course I wondered whether they weren't evidence of an excessive build up (overgrowth) of fungi. Maybe the turmeric didn't agree with them so they'd decided to move along and out?

Once I started the functional medicine doctor's gut treatment (see chapter 8), I again had another health practitioner whom I could ask for advice. So when he asked me how his treatment was going I naturally mentioned those unusual blobs which had started making a regular appearance. Immediately he wanted to know which tract they were coming from. When he learnt that it was my GI tract, he simply shrugged it off. Again I was left none the wiser. But he did reassure me that turmeric was very good as the active ingredient curcumin had many beneficial properties. However, I didn't need to continue with it as his gut treatment would take over the process of rectifying the imbalance in my gut between good and bad microorganisms.

3.Gut dysbiosis

The functional medicine doctor's detoxification treatment had targeted the unhealthy state that my gut was in. He'd introduced me to the terms "dysbiosis" and "microbiome", by explaining that disease causing pathogens were overwhelming the beneficial microbes in my gut. I learnt that the integrity of my gut wall had been damaged by excessive pressure, but apparently in addition the mucosal epithelial barrier (intestinal lining) had been further weakened by dysbiosis. There were simply far too many nasty pathogens in my belly as they were outnumbering the helpful bacteria.

The detox treatment continued the good work turmeric had started. I'd noticed what looked to me like fungi being expelled, so I had no doubt that excessive quantities of noxious organisms had adhered to the epithelial surface of my gut. Once they'd been dislodged they needed to be replaced with good bacteria, which is what the probiotic supplements would've accomplished. The aim was to reduce available gut wall space for pathogens. I'm convinced that by early August 2011 a healthy habitat for good bacteria had been created in my gut.

To ensure my gut microbiome remained with a healthy ratio of pathogens to beneficial bacteria I also continued to follow the advice in Dr Crook's book that encouraged a low-sugar diet to reduce yeast colonisation in the gut. His opinion was that fungal overgrowth would have a negative effect on immune function.

When I'd asked the functional medicine doctor for his opinion of Dr Crook's theory he'd not dismissed the ideas outright as another doctor had done. Instead he'd simply said that the book was getting dated. The advantages of vitamin A had been discussed in connection with improving the structural integrity of mucosal cells, but since then the significant role vitamin D3 plays in regulating the immune system had been recognised by scientists.

Towards the end of the decade further medical research into curcumin also began to indicate that it may assist in maintaining the integrity of the endothelial cells that line the circulatory system. As endothelial cells are a type of epithelial cell, I think it would be reasonable for me to infer that the essential ingredient of turmeric may also have helped repair my gut's epithelium (intestinal lining). Maybe microscopic lesions that would've been the result of faecal impaction repaired themselves and the integrity of my gut was restored.

Eventually I realised that the functional medicine philosophy of "treating the root causes of disease" where possible was aligned with the beliefs of Campbell and Crook. Like Integrative Medicine practitioners, a "differential diagnosis" may be made based on the possibility that many contributing factors could underly a patient's illness. Like my GP this doctor was open-minded. They were both aware of the vast amount of clinical observations that've accumulated over millennia. Exact mechanisms may not yet have been proven through extensive and rigorous randomised, double-blind, placebo controlled clinical trials. However, they knew from experience that the alternative treatments they offered to their patients worked. In the case of the functional medicine doctor who successfully treated my dysfunctional gut, his knowledge was even based on personal experience. These doctors have no option but to become "cross-over" doctors. In other words they have a foot in both camps; modern medicine, and alternative medicine where many ideas/methods have come from ancient medical traditions.

4.Nutritional deficiencies

More than two years on from when things first started going wrong I'd certainly grown older, but also a lot wiser and healthier. Many lessons had been relearned and I'd received advice from numerous health practitioners. However, the straightforward guidelines I'd obtained from Campbell's book in 1997 remained in the forefront of my mind; viz.

- Nutrition
- Elimination
- Circulation

Towards the end of 2011 I'd formulated my own "Preventative Treatment Plan" which Dr Singh had updated in November of that year (see chapter 15). By then I knew that vital nutrients, such as Vitamin D3, strengthened the immune system and helped stop infective microbes from having free reign. Of course, a nutrient rich diet also supported the immune system. But I asked myself:

"What if some key essential vitamins and trace minerals for one reason or another were missing?"

It's known that as we age our immune system flags. As my precious daughter had lovingly informed me, I was heading for my 65th birthday; the age that some clinical guidelines use to mark the beginning of the "elderly" age bracket. Would it be best to err on the side of caution? After checking the Harvard School of Health's website my decision was determined as it stated:

"Each stage of the body's immune response relies on the presence of many micronutrients."

Vitamins C & D were identified as critical for the growth and function of immune cells. These cells that are part of our innate immune system will go into bat for us and attack foreign microbes that manage to enter our bodies. I felt I needed to use whatever means were available to boost my immune system; to protect myself from future "infective problems".

Apparently, our adaptive immune system also needs an immune modulator like Vit D. This is why scientists are researching the associations between vitamin D deficiency and "so-called autoimmune diseases" like rheumatoid arthritis.

To reduce the chance of key nutritional gaps occurring I decided to largely stick with my "Preventative Treatment Plan":

Cod Liver oil (vitamins A & D)

Vitamins D3, C & B3

Multivitamin & Trace Minerals

Besides my trusty tip from Campbell's book (a daily tablespoon of Cod Liver oil), the other supplements had been recommended by specialists; viz. microbiologist, cardiologist and dermatologist.

In addition to these key vitamins, I still stuck rigidly to the "hunter-gatherer" diet throughout 2012.

5.Weight & SAD (Standard Australian Diet)

Current conventional medical wisdom is that there's no such thing as an "Arthritis Diet" that will provide a cure. Of course this is understandable as there are many different types of arthritic disease. However, in my case I think a healthy, balanced diet equates with a healthy gut diet. As such its role is part and parcel of My Concept and could contribute to correcting both chronic constipation and inflammation associated with a weak immune system.

I think poor food choices were a precursor to the health issues that I eventually experienced. A little over a decade ago, when I moved with Peter to a mining town in regional WA, I'd let myself slide into unhealthy eating habits. After an annual health check I'd been given confronting news. I was prediabetic and if I didn't correct my diet there could be serious consequences. This very soon saw me attending dietary information courses at the local, country hospital. At the end of the dietician's presentation she'd suggested I purchase one of the books on display at the back of the room.

- Brand-Miller, J. and others, 2002: *The new glucose revolution; to achieve weight loss, blood glucose control and life-long health with GI*, Hodder, Sydney, Australia.

To encourage me she added that if I put my mind to it my prediabetic condition could be completely reversed. All I needed to do was correct my unhealthy eating habits which were SAD; i.e. typical of the Standard Australian Diet that caused obesity.

From that day forward my diet steadily evolved in a positive direction. By the time I received the Claremont naturopath's advice to follow a "hunter-gatherer" diet (see chapter 6), I'd already dropped a few seriously delicious, but awfully bad habits. One of the worst was my regular evening treat; a generous bowl of Connoisseur gourmet ice cream topped with a good drizzle of Penfolds port. What was I thinking!

My strict low-sugar diet in 2012 meant I began to habitually avoid modern, white refined-carbs and processed foods that are often loaded with sugar. Delicious sugary pastries ceased to tempt me. By 2013 I'd shed 6 kgs and hopefully prevented *C. albicans* from regaining a dominant presence in my gut.

Fortunately, my diet today is still very different from what I got into the habit of carelessly consuming. When a cardiologist encouraged Peter to follow a diet consisting of an abundance of fresh whole fruit and vegies, it became even easier for me to never stray back to old, harmful habits. This heart specialist also supported a low-sugar diet. Apparently, Britain's journal *Nature* had published a paper on the dangers of sugar. The toxic effects of sugar then became a popular topic on ABC radio, which led me to purchase another book that proved to be a fascinating read.

- Gillespie, D., 2008: *Sweet Poison...why sugar makes us fat,* Penguin Books, Melbourne, Australia.

These days my diet could be described as "flexitarian", with hardly any red meat, and fish or chicken only once or twice a week. Each morning I eagerly kick-start the day with an apple and blueberry fruit salad, laced with oats, topped with yoghurt and a generous garnish of pepitas and sunflower seeds. It's a bowl jam-packed with nutrients, antioxidants, prebiotics and probiotics.

6.Bone density and ageing

"Just pump me full of cortisone and I'll be alright."

What I'd asked a rheumatologist to do in 1997 still rings in my years. Its evidence of how distressed I was by what was happening to my body. Overnight I'd begun to hobble. The fear of losing my mobility was very real.

Thanks to fine doctors both in 1997 and again in 2011, I narrowly avoided going down the harmful path of corticosteroid injections. It's my belief that ongoing corticosteroid therapy could've wreaked havoc in my body. In the first instance my immune response would've been suppressed, just when it was most needed to protect my body from harmful invaders. Worse still it would've exacerbated the leaching of calcium from my bones.

I only came to fully understand the rheumatologist's reluctance in late 2012 when I again consulted Jenner's book. By then I was familiar with OA, the diagnosis I'd been given. Simple curiosity prompted me to read the sections on RA and Ank Spond too, as those conditions had been on the radar more than a decade before.

What I read made me shudder:

"Powerful corticosteroids can cause [serious] side effects, including an increased risk of osteoporosis."

There were other unwanted side effects too, such as weight gain and raised blood sugar. Truly I felt as though I'd dodged a bullet, particularly as I sensed I could be genetically predisposed to osteoporosis.

When my mother, whom I adored, had passed away suddenly in 1995 I'd been grief stricken. The moment I last heard her voice was one evening when the phone rang unexpectantly while I was on duty at the Notre Dame Library's desk. I'd eagerly told my Mum how I looked forward to showing her the charming Freo University campus where I worked. But sadly it was not to be.

Within 3 days I was on a plane with my brother flying to Melbourne. The day after the surprise phone call, my mother had been hit by a car while crossing High Street; something she simply shouldn't have done. The impact wasn't severe, but the consequences were disastrous. You see her skeleton at the age of 83 was unbelievably brittle. There were multiple fractures which she wouldn't survive.

As the years passed I'd noticed my Mum shrinking. I'd not paid much heed as I assumed it was a consequence of ageing. By the time she reached 80 her spine had curved and formed a dowager's hump.

So as 2012 drew to a close and with only one final appointment at the Hollywood specialist centre remaining, I again drew up a list of questions for Dr Golledge. As usual he was open and helpful and he'd swiftly responded to my request for a Bone Mineral Density (BMD) test.

The diagnosis of osteopenia that I received at my final appointment for the year with my GP wasn't surprising. Ostelin, a calcium and vitamin D3 supplement was added to my little collection of brekky supplements.

Ageing and the associated decline in my immune function would hopefully be reduced by my nutrient-rich preventative treatment plan. What I also hoped to avoid was to follow in my mother's footsteps. If possible I'd maintain the strength in my bones. I wanted to continue to stand tall and erect; I certainly didn't want to rapidly shrink.

7.Deleterious lifestyle choices: Aerobic exercise, Alcohol & Sleep

Towards the end of 2013 I was no longer mystified by doctors' references to my immune system, as a robust response was needed to counter pathogenic invaders and deal with any "infective problems". However, they also all recommended aerobic exercise; what form, was the question.

"Lots of huffing and puffing" was Dr Singh's recommendation; his young colleague had mentioned hydrotherapy, high-intensity resistance training was discussed in Phelp's tome, Lam's book enthused about the benefits of Tai Chi, while Campbell warned that,

"a decreased lack of exercise could lead to stagnation of toxins within the muscles and joints."

In the end I decided that my exercise program of choice needed to be sustainable; an activity I thoroughly enjoyed that would increase blood circulation.

For me brisk walking was the answer, however the problematic issues of hobbling and a sailor's peg-leg gait had to first be dealt with. In 1997 elimination and ginkgo biloba, the ancient Chinese medicine used to improve circulation, had almost instantly restored normal mobility. Second time around in 2011 my awkward gait, excruciating hip pain and throbbing knee, had needed modern medical therapies. Macrodantin and voriconazole had come to the rescue.

As I no longer experienced any form of pain, continuing to keep the "pain record" that had been recommended in Jenkin's book was pointless. I decided instead to follow Campbell's suggestion and started a "walking record". Fortunately the heart attack-like pains (costochondritis) had also ceased thanks to voriconazole (see chapter 23), so Peter and I began to embark on more extended walks along the banks of the Swan. We were both thrilled with the results. Once or twice I even accompanied Peter all the way along Mounts Bay Road to his office in the CBD.

Choosing brisk walks along the banks of a river teeming with bird life, the occasional dolphin and active people participating in regattas had benefits beyond basic circulation. Such enjoyable walks in the cool, afternoon sea-breeze soothed my soul and as a result would've also boosted my immune system. As the lovely lady GP trained in traditional Chinese medicine had said:

"Western medicine helps us not to die. Eastern medicine teaches us how to live."

My walks were a form of therapy that provided a reprieve from the occasional daily stressors of life. Often they contribute to good, sound sleep too.

At the height of my painful attacks and ensuing anxiety, restful sleep became a thing of the past. The feedback from some doctors left me confused and perplexed. Particularly unhelpful was being asked, "What about the pain?"(see chapter 3). This distressed me as once the attacks ceased there was no pain. However, I was firmly told by some in early 2011, that the painful attacks would be ongoing. All I could do was rely on myself and the signals, or in my case the lack of signals, that my body sent me. Naturally this anxiety further disturbed my sleep.

Undeterred, I looked for a solution to my disrupted sleep pattern and found it between the covers of a book by Jordan Peterson:

- Peterson, J., 2018: *12 Rules for life; an antidote to chaos,* Penguin Random House, UK.

He talked about uncertainty and how this could interfere with sleep cycles. He even mentioned how such stress and tension could "shut down one's immune system". This was something I had already gained an understanding of thanks to Dr Singh (see chapter 20).

According to Peterson,

"Waking up at a consistent hour is a necessity, as negative emotions are tightly tied to disturbed cyclical rhythms."

It didn't take long before I'd restored a regular sleep routine, so regular in fact that my 6am alarm eventually simply wasn't needed. Quite naturally I started surfacing at dawn along with our garrulous family of kookaburras.

But still, I feel I ought to confess, a 6am alarm was just a part of my sleep routine; the best and utterly seductive bit begins the night before. At 10pm once I'm reassured by the sound of Peter's quiet snoring, I dim the lights and turn up the volume; soft, easy listening orchestral music is my favourite. This pre-bedtime interlude comes with a nightly glass of crisp SSB. It's a little wickedness that started many years ago on the recommendation of my GP at the time. I know it's a bad habit and I have good intentions of stopping one day. However, this regular routine does ensure a sound 7 hour slumber and helps maintain my immune system, because according to the Harvard website:

"Sleep is a time of restoration for the body, during which a type of cytokine is released that fights infection."

CONCLUSION:

In July 2013 I'd had a lot to celebrate; not just my 60th birthday, but all my health achievements too (see Figure 10). I'd completed follow-up checks with Doctors Singh, Brennan and Golledge. My GP together with the gastroenterologist and microbiologist, had given me the "all clear".

To receive the positive feedback that my whole body was in good working order had been immensely reassuring. My doctors had given me a strong sense of certainty which prompted me to draw up a list of goals:

- Maintain a strong immune system to help avoid future infections/inflammation
- Stop/minimise the possibility of harmful "infective" inflammation episodes recurring
- Continue to protect all the joints in my body from erosive attacks by implementing primary preventative measures
- Reduce the loss of calcium from my skeleton to help maintain an erect posture
- Remain fit, active and pain free by slowing/stopping both arthritis and osteoporosis
- Assist a healthy immune response (that would decline with age) by ensuring against nutritional deficiencies
- Adopt necessary lifestyle changes to avoid premature ageing

With calm confidence I looked forward to the years ahead. The seemingly endless list of questions that had been in the forefront of my mind were mostly answered.

So, were my goals utterly fanciful? Come 2021, ten years on from when health issues (including arthritis) surfaced, I would revisit the specialists who'd stepped up and helped me. I would obtain as much concrete evidence as I could to support My Concept regarding "arthritis and the gut connection".

Chapter 25 MY PAIN, SENSATIONS & DISCOMFORT (2014)

Once my primary prevention plan was in place there was no longer a need for frequent check-ups with my GP; particularly as I was fit and active. In January with my annual 2014 health tests completed I briefly considered dropping my arthritis research project. However, the "ongoing wear and tear" opinion that I'd been given in 2011 for OA in my right hip continued to puzzle me; the question in the forefront of my mind was:

Why am I totally pain free?

Three years had passed since the start of my arthritis story and Dr Singh had become not just my GP, but also my advisor regarding lifestyle choices and stress management. As I appreciated his wise counsel, I'd told him how I would miss my regular check-ups now that my health issues had been resolved. To my surprise he'd replied:

"You may not be in any pain, but you still have an issue with your right hip. I suggest we do another MRI review midway through this year."

In 2011 some doctors had held the opinion that I urgently needed a total hip replacement, but in 2012 Dr Golledge had assured me this was no longer the case. Apparently, it would be up to me to decide whether or not to have surgery. This was a daunting decision as a total hip replacement was a significant operation. Without any pain or discomfort how was I to know when to make the non-trivial decision to have major surgery?

Of course, in the back of my mind was the functional medicine doctor's statement that my "condition could be stabilised" (see chapter 8). For the previous three years this certainly appeared to have been the case and yet I'd heard another health practitioner disparagingly comment that such doctors "were not to be trusted as they were a bit wacky. They made money by claiming they could 'cure' arthritis, when actually all they were doing was treating an infection." What became an additional concern for me was that if I continued to trust the functional medicine doctor's encouraging prognosis, would some people consider me foolishly optimistic, even a bit touched?

Informed decision making

By 2014 I'd become accustomed to receiving conflicting opinions from medical practitioners, which had left me confused. So I also landed up collecting advice and information from friends who could speak from personal experience. One evening over dinner with a group of friends at our home I plucked up the courage to ask:

"Do you think I'm risking doing further damage to my hip joint by delaying surgery?"

Their responses were truly surprising and just as conflicting as the doctors had been. In summary I discovered that there wasn't a close correlation between apparent damage on radiographic images and actual arthritic symptoms that patients experienced. Another friend told me she'd decided against surgery as a physiotherapist had restored function in her knee. However, it was the story that Kent related which really made us all sit up and pay attention. What he told us was extraordinary and he generously offered to send me a copy of his "ulcer experiences" to use in this book. It's the story of "an infective problem" a bit like mine.

Kent's Ulcer Timeline

The very next day the following email appeared in my inbox.

"Hi Mary Anne,

This is a rough timeline as some of the dates are lost in time.

In 1967 (16 years old) I had unexplained stomach pains. Then in 1969 I returned early from vacation work experience in Tasmania after having stomach pains; nearly fainting while working underground. I underwent test work by taking a Barium Meal during Xrays and I was diagnosed with a duodenal ulcer. Medical advice was it was caused by excessive stomach acid which in turn was caused by stress. A surgical solution was offered which involved cutting the vagus nerve to the stomach (vagotomy). I rejected this idea as I never considered I was a stressful person and could not believe there was that much wrong with me (self-confidence instilled by my mother and father).

During summer vacation employment at Mt Isa in 1971 I passed out one morning and struck my face on the side of a wall. The deep cut in my upper lip did not bleed which caused concern. I went to Mount Isa Base Hospital and received stitches, had blood tests and blood transfusions, and spent several days in hospital until there was no blood in my stools. From that point on I learned to manage stomach pain by drinking milk.

After graduating I worked in Kalgoorlie and Mount Isa. Then my first professional engineering role was in Tennant Creek. While there in 1977 I had another episode when I vomited blood one morning at work. I was flown to Alice Springs after I was given plasma in the RFDS aeroplane and had blood transfusions in Alice Springs Hospital.

In 1977, or thereabouts, I was prescribed a new drug, Tagamet, which is a stomach acid inhibitor, which managed the symptoms quite well.

Around the mid-1980s Dr Wally Kazmarczyk, my GP, said one of his colleagues, Dr Barry Marshall, was seeking patients to participate in clinical trials of antibiotic treatment. His theory was that "ulcers were caused by bacterial infection damaging the protective mucous lining of the gut resulting in gastric ulcers". I was managing the symptoms with Tagamet so I declined to participate in the trial. But in 1990 when the trials were proven successful, I took the course of multiple antibiotics which completely killed the bacteria.

All fixed after 23 years with no recurrence.

Good luck!

Regards,

Kent

As I read Kent's story I felt a surge of gratitude. He'd swept away concerns that my ideas were daft. Instead, it dawned on me that not only could doctors be fallible, but occasionally the entire medical establishment could get things wrong. This good friend had strengthened my resolve to complete my 10-year study of a sample of one.

Characteristic arthritic gaits

Soon after our dinner party I happened to pass by our local chemist and noticed the pharmacist wasn't his usual sprightly self. He was noticeably walking with difficulty, so I decided to raise the topic of my hip with him. Like others he too was very forthcoming with helpful information. He openly shared his health problem with me, saying he'd already lined up a time at the Hollywood Hospital nearby to have his hip replaced. Naturally I shared my situation with him and explained that I too faced a decision regarding a hip replacement. Immediately he reassured me saying that orthopaedic surgeons carried out THR operations frequently and such operations enjoyed a very high success rate. But then he did add a word of caution, advising me to choose a surgeon who was experienced.

As I headed out the door the pharmacist called me back. He'd been observing my gait, much like the doctors had done. The feedback he gave me was greatly reassuring as all he could detect was a barely noticeable limp. Don't worry he laughingly said:

"You don't have a Trendelenburg gait like mine."

If he'd seen me in April 2011 his response would've been very different as back then I'd "walked like a sailor" (see chapter 5), and later developed a peg-leg/stick-like gait. I realised that the manner in which I'd managed to rehabilitate myself was actually rather astonishing.

A few weeks later I attended a business function with Peter and I'm ashamed to say I found myself surreptitiously observing another unusual gait. An elderly man had difficulty raising his foot when he stepped forward. As luck would have it this amiable gentleman chose to come and sit beside me. I don't remember how it came about, but we too landed up discussing hip replacements. Before long I'd gained two more pieces of information which would help with my decision making later in the year. He revealed that a deep nerve had been severed during his THR operation. Like the pharmacist he stressed the importance of choosing a surgeon with years of experience. He even made a few suggestions. But how was I to know when to make such a decision? To this he gave me a helpful tip:

"Don't worry, you'll know when the time comes. It'll start to get you every time you stand up. I wouldn't wait 'til you find yourself crawling with pain."

He also predicted that the distance I could comfortably walk would slowly but surely decrease.

Objective measures that index levels of arthritic pain

With all this talk of doom and gloom, doubt started to creep into my thoughts. Maybe I was just super resilient and could endure pain that others buckled under? Had my optimism induced a powerful placebo effect?

Around Easter time in 2014 I'd begun to think that the amiable gentleman's prediction regarding walking distances might just be materializing. The change was ever so subtle; I first noticed it while I was shopping for Lindt bunnies. Instead of my usual long strides that had helped me keep up with Peter on our Matilda Bay walks, my steps became less free and easy. But ... there was still no pain. This made me think that what I needed was an objective means of assessing whether the damage in my right hip was progressing. I needed a tool which I could use to measure any trends.

Back in 2011 not long after my severe arthritis attack I'd visited the Arthritis Foundation's bookshop where I'd found some informative texts and self-help booklets. Along with the free booklets I'd been given a leaflet advertising a wide range of talks, seminars and workshops. "Pain management strategies" and "How to cope with pain and fatigue" were mentioned. Over the two years prior to 2014 I'd not felt the need to avail myself of all these opportunities. However, given the subtle changes I'd noticed I began attending lectures at the centre; sessions that were often free of charge.

It was at one of these seminars that I learnt about two methods that had been devised by universities to measure not just arthritic pain, but also a person's ability to function and carry out normal, daily tasks.

- The Oxford Hip Score
- The WOMAC OA Index

A third classification scheme used by rheumatologists and radiologists was also mentioned.

- Kellgren-Lawrence Radiographic Classification of OA

Armed with three different methods that were used by doctors to grade arthritic severity I felt a sense of reassurance that my decision whether or not to have THR surgery could be made with more certainty.

The collapse of "wind-sock shaped paralabral cyst"

For three years my success at rehabilitating myself and remaining free of any form of pain or discomfort made me think that maybe ...

just maybe ... I'd truly avoided hip surgery. Sadly though, it was this overconfidence that ultimately became my undoing.

Back in November 2011 when the visiting trainee surgeon from the UK had examined me, she'd paid close attention to the ease with which I moved (see chapter 16). It was significant that I'd simply stood on one leg and then the other when dressing, much like a fit young person would do. I felt this contributed to the surgeon's decision that surgery could be postponed. From then on I prided myself in my ability to drag on jeans quickly and easily.

But one morning in early May 2014 something gave way in my hip. I felt the femur slip and heard a bit of a crunch, but there was no pain whatsoever. Nevertheless, it was rather disconcerting, and it did make me wonder what had happened inside my hip joint. I recalled the radiologist's descriptions of damaged cartilage and wondered whether a labral tear had given way. Could I now be at risk of the ball slipping out of the socket?

Even though I was still not in any pain I decided it would be wise to follow Dr Singh's advice and get another MRI scan done of my hip.

Evidence from radiographic images and my Oxford Hip Score

Before my MRI review appointment with my GP, Peter and I discussed whether we thought a hip operation was on the cards. We both knew I didn't experience any pain and that I could still get out and about. My walking speed may have slowed ever so slightly, but that was all. Neither of us were keen on the idea of major hip surgery, but on the off chance that Dr Singh might refer me back to an orthopaedic surgeon to have my "condition managed", we decided to complete the Oxford Hip Score. The result was encouraging as it suggested moderate hip arthritis; apparently "surgical intervention might not be likely."

With this knowledge I optimistically anticipated a similar result from the radiologists' grading system. The Kellgren-Lawrence Radiographic Classification consists of five categories:

- 1. No OA; 2. Doubtful; 3. Mild; 4. Moderate; 5. Severe.

The MRI report in June 2011 had placed me in the mild-moderate category and attention had been drawn to "a degenerative labral tear and a wind-sock shaped paralabral cyst". Knowing my Oxford score I anticipated a similar result from the scan. But sadly, what my May 2014 MRI showed was that:

"In the near 3 year interval, there has been substantial progression in right hip osteoarthritis, which is now severe."

Possibly if it wasn't for my less alarming Oxford Hip Score, Dr Singh may well have encouraged me to see a surgeon then and there. But instead he chose to explain the deterioration that had occurred over the 3 year interval. He drew my attention to the fact that the radiologist had specifically followed up on the "paralabral cyst", which was no longer there as the hollow remnant had collapsed. This explained the slippage and crunch that I'd felt and heard. He went on to reassure me that my hip joint was stable thanks to my strong muscles and ligaments which were not damaged. There was little chance of my hip dislocating.

Referred pain

With my confidence only slightly dented following the GP's appointment I carried on regardless and began looking forward to an extra special occasion. My July 14th birthday was coming up and our adult children had spoilt me with a gift voucher for a degustation dinner. Bastille day arrived and we headed out in the evening to celebrate along with the French. Living close to the city centre it didn't take long before Peter and I were comfortably settled in a cosy corner of the restaurant. The molded, curved chairs provided plenty of support which was good as we were kept entertained with a steady supply of delicious delicacies right up until midnight.

With the arrival of the bewitching hour came a weird turn of events. Instead of hopping up with Peter and heading for the door I remained momentarily frozen; unable to stand up. The scooped shape of the chair had somehow impacted on my hip joint. Not wanting to distress my dear man I landed up awkwardly standing by using the power of my left leg only. The right remained bent and when it came to straightening it the pain was extreme ... but it wasn't my hip, it was my knee! It immediately dawned on me that this was what the amiable gentleman had implied when he'd warned: "It'll start to get you every time you stand up."

The very next day another appointment was made with Dr Singh and unsurprisingly a fresh MRI scan was organised. My GP didn't think there was anything wrong with my knee; the severe pain had been referred from my hip.

Decision to have surgery

I finally returned to discuss surgery with Dr Witherow, who didn't waste time and got straight to the point. He told me my OA was now very advanced with almost complete loss of joint space, which meant that basically my right hip's cartilage had almost completely disintegrated. I realized that with bone wearing on bone the ball of the femur would be subjected to further damage and further bone loss would occur in the hip socket.

Of course, I was now confronted with a clear understanding of what the functional medicine doctor had meant when he'd bluntly stated: "We can't repair." But then to my surprise I was given some very encouraging additional feedback. The MRI in October 2014 had been more extensive than the one 5 months earlier. In addition to my right hip, my pelvic girdle had also been scanned. Unlike my right hip my "left hip joint space [was] preserved and adequate." This was really good news. It meant that the cartilage in my left hip was fine; it's role as a buffer ensured there was adequate space between the head (ball) of my femur and the acetabulum (socket).

A hip replacement procedure is significant surgery, but I'd run out of options as I'd used practically all nonsurgical therapies. In my case a total hip replacement (THR) was the option of last resort. Corticosteroid medications could've provided temporary relief but knowing the associated severe side effects I certainly wasn't going to go down that path. Briefly in November a walking stick had temporarily restored my reduced mobility, but when I began using my supermarket trolley as a walker I decided to focus on preparing myself for surgery.

Along with a set date for my THR came a substantial information booklet from the Hollywood Hospital. Adjacent to the hospital was a well set up gym staffed with physiotherapists. I availed myself of this facility by booking sessions both pre and post op. By the time the 9th December 2014 arrived I felt confident I was physically and mentally prepared.

My conscientious determination paid off, but I know my experienced surgeon also had a major part to play in my swift recovery. To this day I can hear the delighted surprise expressed by the nurses when they'd changed my dressing the day after the operation. In unison they'd cooed: "Oh my, but that's beautiful!" Today all I have to indicate that I now have a titanium and ceramic hip is a barely visible fine line; not a stitch mark in sight ... they weren't needed.

Conclusion

Within less than four weeks post my THR I felt as good as new. The operation had been a success and it very effectively provided symptomatic relief. However, I didn't allow myself to slip into complacent bad habits. Instead, I reminded myself that the THR had managed my hip problem. It wasn't preventative or curative treatment.

The doctors who'd stepped up and provided treatment for underlying causes were not forgotten and it pleased me to find that they'd not forgotten me either. As I was surfacing from my anaesthetic induced slumber post-op I was startled to see Dr Golledge appear in the recovery ward. Through the haze I recognised his warm smile as he gave my shoulder a reassuring squeeze, saying "You've done it now. It's over."

But was it? I was to discover that there were naysayers to contend with; those who dismissed as fanciful the notion that I'd managed to stabilise my arthritis. In my usual pig-headed fashion I made a commitment to myself. I would persist and complete my 10-year study of a sample of one.

Chapter 26 POST THR (2015)

At the start of 2015 I knew I'd completely recovered and in record time too. I was buoyed with optimism and looked forward to enjoying activities with my grandchildren in the gardens of UWA. Yet sadly I seemed to be surrounded by cynics; after all I was no longer a spring chicken and many considered arthritis to be an old person's disease. Their scepticism left me a bit subdued and damaged my self-confidence. Was I chasing a false hope, a fantasy?

My confidence was further dented when I read an article in *The Australian* about Jane Fonda. The interview with this iconic actress from my era frankly discussed body issues and ageism. In the '80s I'd enthusiastically followed her *Workout Challenge* video in an effort to emulate the agile and fit beauty. Alas in 2015 she openly admitted that her "body hurt almost all the time." At 77 instead of running she walked and her workouts were "slow"; yoga was too hard. This magnificent role model had "got arthritis"; her skeleton now had a lot of metal in it ... fake knee, fake hip, fake bits in her spine. I was led to wonder whether a similar fate lay in store for me.

Still, I wasn't going to allow myself to get miserable. Instead, Peter helped by ferrying me to my rehabilitation appointments at the hospital gym. In addition the physio provided me with exercises to keep up at home, all of which must've helped my speedy recovery and soon I began looking forward to catching up with friends.

Prevailing lay opinions regarding my arthritis

Parking where we live is limited at the best of times but given the huge amount of construction underway up the road at the time, finding parking at the Hollywood Hospital could be impossible. Understandably patients like me had been asked to discourage ward visitors. So come January 2015 a small group of friends contacted me, eager to drop by to see how I was faring. Ever since I'd procrastinated and delayed hip surgery for close to four years there'd been raised eyebrows. What was I thinking following my own course?

When the sceptics gathered in our lounge-room for coffee I immediately found their attention was focussed on me. One at a time they launched into providing me with unsolicited, gratuitous medical advice. The leader began by edging forward on the sofa opposite me saying,

"We're very concerned about you. Please tell us how is your leg?"

In an attempt to diffuse the uncomfortable situation I laughingly responded:

"Oh Cyn ... I have to be so careful otherwise it might fall off!"

The others almost collapsed with laughter, but Cyn did not. Instead she reprimanded me.

"No ... I asked you nicely."

With absolute honesty I then explained that I'd recovered from my THR op in record time. The physio at the Hollywood hospital had me standing just four hours post-op and doing set exercises in the gym the following day. I had been good to go home in record time.

Quietly I thought that if this didn't allay their concerns then what would?

But then Cyn's friend became mildly distressed. She turned towards me and clutched my hands while saying beseechingly,

"You do realise you're going to have to have your other hip replaced too."

All I could do was shrug and calmly reply,

"Well, I guess we'll just have to wait and see."

Understandably this weird scenario left me feeling mildly disturbed, so I raised the question with Dr Singh at my annual check-up saying,

"Even though I feel as good as new and Peter describes me 'like a sprightly gazelle on steroids', I'm left questioning myself. Do you believe I'm thinking clearly?"

My dear GP lent forward and rested his hand lightly on my wrist.

"Look my dear, it's easy to see whether someone's crazy. You're definitely not crazy. You're thinking very clearly."

Nevertheless, I wondered about the functional medicine doctor's promise that he would stabilise my arthritis. Thankfully my doctor came up with a practical solution.

"You will have three review appointments with Dr Witherow this year. In December he'll arrange for a repeat x-ray of your pelvic girdle. Why don't you request that the radiologist does a comparison with last year's images?"

Review appointments post-surgery

Less than 6 weeks post-op I walked crutch-free up a steep city street towards the beautiful Wesley Uniting Church Chapel to attend my nephew's wedding to his petite Thai sweetheart. Had Dr Witherow been watching he would've been pleased. With my first review appointment coming up I started jotting down points that I wished to raise with him to make sure I was well informed and able to counter the pessimism of cynics.

I decided to leave the question of whether my arthritis had been stabilised to later in the year as front of mind was the possibility of hip implant failure. Unpleasant stories of such occurrences had been circulating, particularly in 2011 (see chapter 16). At that time cobalt particles flaking off prosthetic hips had produced deleterious consequences. There'd also been talk of the possibility that the cement fixative around the stem of the prosthesis could weaken; it wouldn't hold forever.

It turned out that those concerns of mine were unwarranted. Dr Witherow had received the physio's report and immediately complemented me on my progress. He was agreeably surprised to discover I'd regained all physical functions. To have achieved 100% rehabilitation in less than four weeks was unusual; even my walking speed was above the norm.

Then to reassure me that he'd implanted a first class prosthesis he gave me a ceramic-on-polyethylene ball and socket implant to hold as he pointed out improvements that had been made saying,

"The cement will hold and the plastic liner shouldn't wear out as the durability has been increased by a factor of ten. These recent improvements mean it should last your lifetime."

Back in 2011 Dr Golledge had told me a hip replacement would last between 15 and 20 years. With quiet delight I realised that procrastinating and delaying my THR had been fortuitous.

As I left, my surgeon gave me an extra compliment but tempered it with caution:

"You're doing exceedingly well, but don't overdo it. I wouldn't run unless you find you have to get out of the way of an oncoming bus!"

Foolishly I didn't take heed. Instead I remembered being told about muscles becoming weak if they weren't used properly. With my rehab sessions at the gym completed I resumed my step-up & step-down exercises at the base of our staircase (see chapter 9). At least I held on firmly to the handrails as I upped the speed of the exercise, but I should have remembered the physio's warning:

"I know you no longer have any physical limitations and don't require pain killers but be cautious as it takes three months for the tissues around your hip joint to knit nice and tight. Up until then there's a slight risk of dislocation."

I paid the price for being overzealous as suddenly my progress slowed when a setback occurred in week 8 post-op. First there was a barely noticeable twinge in my right buttock which increased as I walked. The next day I had to swallow my pride and an endone pain killer, before I headed out the door with a walking stick again in hand.

From then on I erred on the side of caution. I couldn't risk doing further damage as another nephew was getting married and this celebration was going to be in Cape Town. I'd have been bitterly disappointed had a poorly hip prevented me from boarding the flight to South Africa.

By week 12 my more tentative approach had paid off. I'd gradually downgraded from an occasional heavy duty endone, to one or two panamax, to no pain killers at all. Dr Witherow was pleased to hear this good news at my appointment in March, but as he was pressed for time he suggested I discuss my minor setback with a young Scotsman who was working alongside him on a trainee fellowship program.

It was a privilege to have this young surgeon give me his undivided attention as I worked through the questionnaire I'd prepared. He didn't scoff at my ambition to write a memoir, but instead took an interest in what arthritis topics I planned to cover. A question that continued to dog me was the lack of a close correlation between the pain trajectory I'd experienced and the Kellgren-Lawrence Radiographic sliding scale from mild to severe. I also wondered what part the antibiotics and antifungal had played. Then there was the promise I'd been given that my arthritis could be stabilized. At the end of the day the idea that my problems were simply the result of 'wear and tear' just didn't make sense to me.

The young surgeon briefly considered my questions and then gave a response based on what the medical profession knew at that point in time:

"It's hard for us to give a precise explanation as doctors don't know everything about arthritis. We're aware that genetics plays a role, then there's damage caused by trauma and of course there's septic arthritis. But people with septic arthritis are very ill; one antibiotic dose wouldn't clear it. Also infections affect bone quality and the head of your femur was not badly damaged. Maybe you had a mild, sub-clinical infective problem, rather than true septic arthritis. We're not 100% sure, but this recent setback you've had is minor. It's likely you just stretched your internal scar. Don't worry, the ball isn't easily dislodged from the socket. Overall you're doing very well. I'm impressed."

Nine months later I returned to see Dr Witherow for my final review. The orthopaedic practice was as busy as ever with few empty seats in the waiting room. As usual I'd allowed plenty of time, so I didn't mind the brief wait before a chair became available. What I hadn't anticipated was that the surgeon might be running late. Eventually I realized that time was running out on my parking meter; I could land up with an unwelcome fine. On the spur-of-the moment I sprung up, let the receptionist know I would be returning and ran around the corner to feed the meter in a side-street.

I completed my dash in the nick of time as on my return I was summoned. Immediately I blurted out my apologies saying, "I'm so sorry but I had to run round the corner to feed the parking meter." At that moment I realized I'd impulsively ignored the surgeon's advice and I apprehensively waited to be admonished. But instead there was a grin:

"Don't worry, your tissues have healed well. You won't have to take strict precautions forever. You also mustn't worry about the hip implant failing. If you feel something's faulty it could possibly be an infection."

With the mention of a possible infection I just had to ask:

"So instead of OA caused by 'wear and tear' could I describe my condition as *'Post infection erosive arthritis in a single joint'*?"

To this I didn't receive a yes or no answer, but I was told,

"Currently there's a big debate as to whether OA is a primary or secondary condition. OA does occur after an infection, but it's not very common. There is a link, though, between OA and the immune system.

Now to make sure your prosthesis has settled without any issues I'm going to send you upstairs for another scan of your pelvic girdle."

With that I asked if he'd send me copies of the radiologist's reports for December 2014 and 2015. I was walking freely and easily;

even capable of running, so surely the images would show my arthritis had been stabilised in my left hip.

It was as though Dr Witherow guessed what I was thinking, as his parting comment was,

"I don't mind if you write your arthritis memoir, but why don't you come back to see me again in six years' time for a true 'final review'."

The promise of a good news story

Before Christmas 2015 I was able to squeeze in a last appointment for the year with Dr Singh. Naturally I was eager to learn what the follow-up reports from the radiologist contained. His expression told the story as he said,

"Your surgeon says you're doing exceedingly well and the radiologist reports that there's no significant change to your left hip joint."

Was this news too good to be true?

It then amazed me to learn from Dr Singh, who'd treated numerous arthritis cases for more than 30 years, that there were many people with cases similar to mine. Of course he knew I wanted to write my good news story so he went on to suggest that I should,

"Just write your story as it happened. Use your data. I will write a foreword for you to provide a medical perspective."

My arthritis stabilised – concrete evidence from radiographic images

The following day the radiologist's reports arrived in the mail. Of course, I already knew the positive result, but I wanted to see and read it for myself. True enough, just as the functional medicine doctor had predicted, there was "no significant change" to my left hip joint space. Thanks to my record keeping, I was able to refer back to my lever-arch files dated 2011 and 2014. I extracted the five radiologist reports that I'd kept and summarised the OA trajectories for first my right hip and then my left.

R. hip trajectory:

- 20/**6/2011** ... *"**Mild-moderate** right hip osteoarthrosis. Evidence of a degenerative tear and chondral wear progressing"* ... [The thickness of damaged cartilage decreasing ... no sign of repair ... degenerative 'wear and tear' ongoing.]
- 13/**5/2014** ... *"In the near 3-year interval, there has been substantial progression in right hip osteoarthritis, which is now **severe;** extensive full thickness cartilage loss"* **...** [All my walking had probably hastened the breakdown of right hip cartilage. But had it been beneficial for my remaining left hip and my knees?]
- 3/**10/2014**: ... *"**Advanced** right hip OA; almost complete loss of joint space"* ... [My cartilage had been worn away; now bone on bone].

L. hip trajectory:

- 3/**10/2014** ... "**Left hip joint space preserved** and adequate."
- 12/**12/2014 ... "Relatively mild** degenerative change at the left hip."
- 3/**12/2015 ...** "Compared to 12/12/2014 a little narrowing is noted, [but] **no significant change has occurred**."... [No evidence of ongoing cartilage degeneration ... OA stabilised]

The stark contrast between my left and right hips was obvious: "Left hip joint space preserved and adequate;" versus "Substantial progression in right hip osteoarthritis with extensive full thickness cartilage loss."

A stable left hip: The radiographic evidence was clear. For 12 months the OA in my left hip had remained stable; it stayed "relatively mild".

My GP agreed with my surgeon, and like Dr Witherow he'd said to me:

"Now we need to see how you go over the next 5 years. A bigger timeframe will indicate how well you're doing long-term; positive MRI images will also become more significant."

Conclusion

Towards the end of 2015 my left hip cartilage was in good condition as the MRI image showed there was adequate space for the ball of my left femur to continue to move comfortably within the joint socket. All the brisk walking that Dr Singh encouraged had produced no evidence of "wear and tear". Just as he and Dr Campbell had predicted the movement had been beneficial as it improved circulation (see chapter 4). I believe that the exercise had reduced the possibility of toxins accumulating and initiating corrosion of my left hip cartilage.

Dr Golledge had also told me vitamin D3 helped the immune system fight infections. In 2011 he'd mentioned that they were only just learning about its significance. Secure in the knowledge that the preventative step of taking a daily dose of vitamin D3 was now evidence based, I rigidly continued with my daily supplement regimen. I wanted to ensure my immune system remained as robust as possible in order to protect my remaining healthy joints from possible damage.

At the age of 63 I continued to enjoy taking long, pain free strides with Peter on our enjoyable brisk river walks. There was no indication that I was following a progressive and degenerative decline into debilitated old age; no negative evidence on radiographic images and no untoward sensations that I could detect.

Would my arthritis still be in abeyance at the end of the decade as I headed towards 70 years of age? As I'd said to a well-meaning friend at the beginning of the year:

"Well, I guess we'll just have to wait and see."

Chapter 27 ADVANCEMENT IN THE UNDERSTANDING OF OA (2016 – 2017)

My renewed enthusiasm for my arthritis project was almost dashed one morning in 2016 when I caught up with a close friend for brunch. I'm sure she had the best of intentions when she earnestly told me that I didn't really have much of a success story as my right hip had ultimately been replaced. Patiently I explained to her that there is both preventative and curative, as well as symptomatic treatment. I told her my right THR had been very successful, but the relief it brought was symptomatic. So far my left hip remained in good condition and I wanted to see if I could keep it that way. To this she just stared in disbelief as she slowly shook her head. My response was to shrug and drop the subject; far better to gaze out over the ocean and draw in a deep soothing breath of fresh sea air.

Nevertheless, at my next appointment with Dr Singh I found myself explaining how few people believed that I'd achieve anything. Instead most appeared to think my ideas were daft. To this my doctor firmly responded:

"You are not a nutcase. You're highly intelligent; having come this far you should complete your story. Look, you're like a canary in a mine. Your case may attract attention, but a significant number of cases like yours are required for a change to take place in medical understanding. It may take twenty years or more."

In spite of my reality check with my GP it was a daunting prospect to envisage persisting with my project while surrounded by cynics.

Afterall, six years stretched ahead of me before I would return to see Dr Witherow. His parting comment in 2015 had been: "Come back and see me in 2021 for a true 'final review'."

Clarification of my form of arthritis

At my review appointments in 2015 with my experienced surgeon and his Scottish trainee, every effort had been made to provide me with a clearer understanding of what might have brought on the disintegration of my right hip cartilage. My successful THR had very effectively managed the grinding discomfort that started to occur once I reached the severe stage of OA - bone rubbing up against bone in my right hip (see chapter 25). However, I continued to wonder how best to ensure my other joints remained healthy.

Both surgeons agreed there had been some sort of "infective problem"; possibly sub-clinical. This prompted me to read up about the pathophysiology of degenerative joint disease. On the Washington University Medical School's website I discovered that "other forms of arthritis frequently may have OA as the end-stage making differentiation difficult. Typically, OA improves with rest and does not remain symptomatic at night-time."

Excruciating attacks that woke me in the middle of the night had marked the start of my arthritis experience, but after the functional medicine doctor's treatment they ceased (see chapter 8). This made me suspect the end-stage OA in my right hip was the secondary result of another form of arthritis. It also made me again question the original diagnosis given to me in 2011:

"You have osteoarthritis. It's a chronic and degenerative condition caused by wear and tear."

At that time it was stated in the Australian Orthopaedic Association's guide for patients that osteoarthritis (wear and tear largely related to age) was a common [primary] cause of joint damage. Imagine our surprise when in 2016 Peter and I learnt that this diagnosis had recently been thrown out; it was now considered archaic. We were driving south towards Augusta on the south-western tip of Australia when we heard this announcement. Dr Norman Swan was interviewing Professor Hunter on the ABC Health Report.

Immediately I lent forward and turned up the volume. I was stunned to hear Australia's leading authority on OA voicing exactly what I'd instinctively thought and then read in Lane's book which discussed a study of the joints of marathon runners (see chapter 12). 'Wear and tear' together with age weren't plausible explanations for my arthritis. Professor Hunter concurred with Dr Lane, stating that joggers aren't "grinding their knees and hips to dust." Apparently these ideas were:

"... definitely not true; completely false. Good studies have shown that exercise [even] running is helpful in preventing OA. Sedentary people are at greater risk."

The professor went on to admit that allied healthcare professionals, such as physiotherapists and dieticians were under-utilised. When he stated that "an ounce of prevention is a whole lot better than cure", I was delighted. He was validating all that I believed and the approach I'd adopted towards gaining the upper-hand over my arthritic condition. It made me wonder what he would think of the alternative diagnostic label I'd found on an American medical website; viz.

"Post infection erosive arthritis in a single joint"

Pathophysiology of OA cartilage

Once the lengthy but fascinating interview with Professor Hunter came to an end Peter turned to me and said:

"You know I think a lot of people with arthritis would be interested in your story. Don't throw all your hard work away."

I nodded and added,

"Yes, I know but I'm not quite sure what the outcome will be in six years' time."

"That doesn't matter ... write the book!"

The following weekend I tentatively began a rough draft. As a courtesy to Dr Singh he was the first to read it and his positive response made me renew my efforts. It was the start of a much-needed wave of support that came from those close to me. Word started to get out and fellow arthritis sufferers began asking me questions.

Something that I'd found curious also puzzled my best friend Jen who was preparing for a total knee replacement. In her usual down-to-earth manner she asked:

"What happened to the cartilage in my knee? Why don't I have any left?"

Fortunately, thanks to a recent presentation I'd attended at the Arthritis Foundation I was able to give her a basic explanation:

"Well, the cushions of cartilage which enable our joints to move smoothly are rubbery bits; remnants of foetal skeleton that didn't harden into bone. If the integrity of the cartilage is damaged for one reason or another its cohesive fabric becomes compromised and with ongoing use it just starts to fall apart. It doesn't contain blood vessels so it can't quickly repair itself in the same way as a stitched wound does. Living on a farm you probably carried on regardless just getting things done. You see cartilage doesn't contain nerves so you wouldn't have felt it steadily disintegrate."

Seeing Jen's disappointment, I then went on to explain that I'd received treatment that had worked for me. My other joints hadn't been affected; maybe there'd even been some improvement. Instead of a pessimistic diagnosis, a functional medicine doctor had told me that:

"We can stabilise [arthritis], but we can't repair [cartilage]."

Jen took on board my explanation, but there was a lot more she wanted to know. With interest she paged through my first draft and said:

"Well, I'd be very interested to read this when it's finished."

My chat with Jen prompted me to double check the accuracy of my description of what might have resulted in her knee cartilage disintegrating. I found just the explanation I was looking for in *The Merck Manual for Health Care Professionals* under the section on joint disorders:

"Normal joints have little friction with movement and do not wear out with typical use, overuse, or most trauma. Hyaline cartilage is avascular, aneural, and alymphatic. It is 95% water and extracellular cartilage matrix, and only 5% chondrocytes. Cartilage health and function depend on compression and release of weight bearing and use; i.e. compression pumps fluid from the cartilage into the joint space and into capillaries and venules, whereas release allows the cartilage to re-expand, hyperhydrate, and absorb necessary electrolytes and nutrients."

This health manual from the US validated the early advice contained in Campbell's book; viz.

- Circulation

When I'd followed his advice back in 1997 it had seemed counter-intuitive, but it had worked. Then in 2015 I'd obtained concrete evidence from MRIs that Dr Singh had also been right when he'd emphasised the need for "plenty of huffing and puffing".

It was encouraging to have certainty, but the Merk Manual went on to cover the grey area I'd already learnt about. Apparently actual triggers of OA are often unknown. Sometimes cartilage damage begins with "mechanical injury" (trauma), or "transmission of inflammatory mediators from the synovium into cartilage"(inflammation).

My OA had not been caused by 'wear and tear'; rather it was the consequence of some sort of trigger such as trauma or inflammation. Despite this lack of certainty the information on cartilage pathogenesis ended with a glimmer of hope for me as even though cartilage degeneration is considered to be progressive it was stated that:

"occasionally, with no predictability, it stops or reverses."

In my case this appeared to have occurred. The December 2015 pelvic scan showed that arthritis had been stopped in my left hip:

"no significant change [only] a little narrowing noted."

Apparently, some joints do improve if arthritis is caught early enough. I felt a skerrick of optimism which strengthened my determination to persist with my health measures (see chapter 24). There was now the real possibility that in six years' time, at my true 'final review' with Dr Witherow, my pelvic scan might reveal that no significant narrowing had occurred in my left hip between the ball and socket; the

"left hip joint space [would be] preserved and adequate."

Primary and secondary causes of OA

Once I'd heard it confirmed by Professor Hunter that the 2011 Australian Orthopaedic Association's explanation for OA (wear and tear largely related to age) had been rejected, I naturally wondered if they'd come up with a more plausible alternative. Disappointingly I discovered that medical technology hadn't yet been able to provide a clear explanation for the pathogenesis of cartilage. There was still no definitive reason for the underlying cause of cartilage disintegration. As it was still largely undefined, medicine had resorted to stating that the primary cause is unknown (idiopathic).

Even though the primary classification for OA is idiopathic, there are several known secondary causes; e.g.

trauma (mechanical), congenital joint abnormalities (genetic), autoimmune disease (immunologic phenomena), sedentary lifestyle, obesity, inflammation (RA) and infections.

All these conditions can alter cartilage structure and disturb normal joint function. I was fairly certain that my arthritis wasn't a primary, generalised disorder, but a secondary disorder that had affected a particular joint. Only my right hip cartilage had disintegrated; my arthritic condition was unilateral.

The challenge that faced me was to decide which secondary trigger had been the likely cause underlying my cartilage degeneration.

Indeed, wear and tear had occurred but it wasn't the primary cause, rather my arthritis was the consequence of severe damage (pseudo-cysts and tears) that had been done to the joint cartilage. This was why the USA doctor I'd contacted online in 2011 had advised:

"You have a cyst in your inner hip socket. You need to determine the underlying cause of the cyst [to] facilitate treatment. If left untreated, this condition can cause permanent, long-term, joint damage".

Good fortune, luck and dogged determination had enabled me to find effective treatment (see chapter 8). I felt the effectiveness of this treatment pointed to "an underlying cause."

A self-explanatory label for my arthritis

To clarify the confusing explanations and conflicting advice I'd received in 2011, I'd resorted to informing myself about arthritis. By reading extensively, attending information sessions at the Arthritis Foundation, questioning GPs and specialists, I hoped to find a more meaningful explanation. In 2015 the surgeons had obligingly answered all my questions and helped me come to an understanding as to why a clear-cut diagnosis wasn't always possible.

However, I remained unsatisfied with the reductive "wear and tear" reason I'd been presented with in 2011. By 2016 it turned out that my intuition had been correct. Such ongoing erosion didn't inevitably form part of the ageing process. As an alternative to this archaic explanation, I initially came up with the label *"post infection erosive arthritis in a single joint"*. This self-explanatory description was based on the up-to-date information in the Merck Manual.

But even though I felt my positive response to antibiotic and antifungal treatment supported my hypothesis that infection had been a secondary cause of my arthritis, my surgeons remained ambivalent (see chapter 26). As a result I later modified my label to *"erosive arthritis a consequence of subclinical septic arthritis"*.

To find support for my label I combed through the radiologists' reports from 2011 to see if they'd been able to detect anything. This is what I found:

20/6/2011 Mild-moderate right hip osteoarthritis:

... "Evidence for mild hip joint synovitis ... *chondral wear progressing"*

Not understanding the terminology, I then referred to the arthritis-research.com website. Amongst the recent research findings I discovered that instead of subclinical septic arthritis I may well have had *"transient toxic synovitis."*

Apparently "it can be a diagnostic challenge to differentiate between septic arthritis and transient toxic synovitis, a pathologic state that's not completely understood. [But] synovitis is clearly associated with a wide spectrum of infectious agents, and the mechanisms underlying this association are varied and complex. [However] this inflammatory process can be completely resolved with treatment. [Apparently] disorders in the spectrum of autoimmunity can intersect to produce synovitis."

With this newfound knowledge thanks to advances in arthritis research I then modified my arthritis label to:

Erosive arthritis secondary to subclinical septic arthritis &/or transient toxic synovitis.

I think these recent arthritis research findings elucidated what might well have been the underlying cause of the excruciating attacks that I'd experienced in 2011.

Dr Golledge review appointment: January 2017

If I was going to write an arthritis story that might possibly help fellow creaky folk, then I needed to get as many facts straightened out in my head as possible. Dr Singh had been extraordinarily helpful, but an infectious disease specialist like Dr Golledge might be able to tell me a bit more about the "inflammatory mediators" in synovial fluid that were mentioned in the Merck Manual. Presumably these toxic mediators that were involved in joint inflammation were the "infectious agents" referred to in the latest research findings that I'd come across. Back in 2011 there'd been references to *'it'*, but when I'd asked the renowned microbiologist if he could explain to me what was going on he'd apologetically simply said; "I'm afraid we don't really know".

The 'wear and tear' explanation had since been thrown out; there was now talk about infectious mediators; maybe Dr Golledge would be able to fill me in on any recent advances in arthritis research. My GP agreed and with that I was able to make an appointment to again see the infectious disease specialist in January 2017.

It had been several years since I'd last seen this well known specialist so we started by trying to remember just how many years had passed. But then he pulled up my records and reminded me that at an appointment in 2013 I'd seen him about a minor autoimmune issue. At the time he'd been very reassuring saying:

"Lots of people have a very low 'ANA titre'. It's insignificant and of no consequence. It just needs to be monitored along with your thyroid."

When I mentioned that I'd recently discovered how "disorders in the spectrum of autoimmunity can intersect to produce [toxic] synovitis," he quickly brushed my concerns aside.

With that I went on to tell him how the rejection of the old 'wear and tear' explanation had reignited my writing ambitions:

"You see it's such a relief to know that what I instinctively thought in 2011 is actually correct. At times over the last six years I've wondered whether I was out of my mind to refute what some doctors believed. But then deep down I realised the idea of people's joints wearing out as they aged was patently ridiculous, otherwise every man and his dog would be queueing up for joint replacements on their 60th birthdays."

This made Dr Golledge chuckle, but he was laughing with me ... not at me.

I then reminded him of our first meetings in 2011 (see chapter 14). We'd talked about diagnostic treatment and the possibility of getting my case published.

"You know Dr Singh thinks my case might attract attention, but that it may well take twenty years or more before my form of arthritis becomes recognised by mainstream medicine."

"Well, he's right, but I don't think a case like yours will get into *The Lancet*."

"Then what about the BMJ? They publish case histories."

"Mmm, you could try, but it won't be easy."

To this I sighed with disappointment. Would all my determined efforts be wasted and come to naught?

"Surely then I could just write an arthritis memoir ... but I've sensed some are opposed to this idea. Do you think medical matters are best left to doctors to deal with?"

"No, not at all. Look ... here's what I'm going to do. I'm going to state in my report that you wish to write a memoir and that I have no objections."

True to his word his report was waiting for me on Dr Singh's desk when I returned to the Claremont Clinic. This is what my GP then read to me:

"I caught up with Mary Anne today; we were able to go through several of her questions and hopefully my answers will be of help going forward. She is now keen to get all her reports and letters for a memoir that she is going to write. I would have no problem at all with this.

Of course, I am absolutely delighted that she has had such a good result from her hip replacement and of course there is only minimal osteoarthritis in the left hip so with luck she should avoid any further major joint replacement surgery."

This generous specialist had gone above and beyond for me. My appointment with him had provided me with more grist for the mill. I returned home filled with enthusiasm and excitement; eager to continue with my arthritis tale. A story that I hoped would be of help to many others who were looking for answers to unclear and sometimes confusing responses.

Conclusion

For a patient to understand their health condition they need first and foremost to be given an accurate diagnosis; ideally one that is self-explanatory. To be told in 2011 that the source of my problem was ongoing 'wear and tear', had been unhelpful. It suggested that there was little, if anything that I could do about the disease. Thankfully doctors Brennan, Singh and Golledge gave me more definitive advice; viz. boost and maintain my immune system. Dr Singh even went a step further and postulated what were the likely underlying causes of my debilitated immune system. It was opportune that the functional medicine doctor provided exactly the treatment I needed to "stabilise" my arthritis. The help I received from these four doctors was serendipitous; thanks to where I live but also my determination to educate myself and steer my own course. Apparently, there are many people like me who are not as fortunate. In all likelihood they could become victims of the self-fulfilling prophecy that "osteoarthritis is a chronic, degenerative disease that commonly afflicts the elderly."

Chapter 28 OA, RA, INFLAMMATIONS AND AGEING (2018)

The period 2015 to 2018 turned out to be seminal years in the development of My Concept of my arthritic condition. At my review appointments in 2015 with my experienced surgeon and the Scottish trainee, every effort was made to provide me with a clearer understanding of what might have brought on the disintegration of my right hip cartilage. My successful THR had very effectively managed the grinding discomfort that started to occur once bone began rubbing up against bone (see chapter 25). However, I continued to wonder how best to look after my other healthy joints.

In early 2018 I remained alert to any new developments in arthritis research. So, when I received advice from the Arthritis Foundation on an upcoming talk discussing how to manage arthritis at home I decided to attend. What captured my attention was the statement:

"The key to living successfully with Arthritis is to understand your condition and to take control of it as soon as possible."

To put an end to confusing explanations and conflicting advice, I'd extensively researched the arthritis topic and looked for alternative, more meaningful, self-explanatory labels. Instead of OA caused by "wear and tear largely related to age" I initially came up with a condition called *post infection erosive arthritis*. Later I modified the label to a more likely diagnosis; viz. *erosive arthritis secondary to subclinical septic arthritis &/or transient toxic synovitis.*

Arthritis and ageing

However, I still wondered about the idea that my arthritis was part and parcel of ageing. The information I'd gathered from GPs and specialists suggested this was not the case. No, my arthritis issue was related to a weakened immune system. Dr Golledge and I had had a chuckle about this nonsensical notion of active people grinding their joints to dust (see chapter 27). Sensible reasoning made me continue to question this ageist approach and I began to put two and two together.

Why was it that OA had become associated with the elderly, yet 70-year-old marathon runners remained unaffected? Was it simply because they didn't lead a sedentary lifestyle, or was there more to this phenomenon? When my daughter had cautioned me not to continue enthusiastically lifting grandchildren up high for a fulsome hug, I'd decided to investigate this "elderly" label that I'd been assigned (see chapter 24), as instinctively I felt it was inappropriate.

You see in many respects I knew I was almost a clone of my mother, yet she and her two sisters had remained amazingly fit and active well into their eighties. Tucked away in my desk drawer I still kept a beautifully written Christmas card depicting snow covered Naarden. It was from my Tante Dorli sent in her 98th year. Not only is there a family history of longevity, but interestingly none of the sisters were arthritic. To my knowledge their skeletons remained metal free.

Puzzled I searched the American National Institutes of Health website and came across an explanation as to why many health practitioners no longer rely on old clinical guidelines which use,

"chronological age as a convention to refer to a person aged 65 years or more as 'elderly'. [This label can't apply to all 65- year old's because] the ageing process is not uniform across the population due to differences in genetics, lifestyle, and overall health."

To my mind the explanation for arthritis increasing with age lay elsewhere.

As it's known that as we age our immune system flags, I'd taken steps to reduce the associated decline in my immune function by adopting a nutrient-rich preventative treatment plan (see chapter 24). This followed on the advice of four physicians who'd emphasised that a robust immune system was key. For me it provided a means of taking control of my arthritic condition and those excruciating flares that I had experienced in 2010 and 2011.

My pain, inflammations and discomfort trajectory

It was a surprise phone call very late one evening that got me thinking again about all those disturbing, unpleasant sensations that had distressed me in 2011. Barb my friend from uni days must've forgotten about the six-hour time difference between Cape Town and Perth. But I soon realised why; she was in a state of distress:

"There was a moment this afternoon when I just couldn't walk. I don't know what's happening! What did it feel like when you couldn't walk properly?"

"You know I didn't feel a thing," I replied. "Peter was more upset than me as the way I swung my leg out looked so weird. The odd thing was that by the time I got to see a doctor it had fixed itself. Maybe a chip of cartilage had caused an obstruction? Anyway, I was glad I didn't rush off to a surgeon."

"Oh ... my doctor thinks surgery is on the cards for me. He says it's because I'm heading for 70."

"Look, in the past 8 years there's been a shift in the understanding of OA. They now no longer accept the idea that 'wear and tear' is inevitable."

"No ... that doesn't sound right," said Barb flabbergasted. "Are you sure?"

With a sigh I explained that I'd also been told about 'wear and tear', old age and wheelchairs in 2011, but thanks to a doctor in the USA I'd been encouraged to find treatment for the underlying cause which wasn't wear and tear, but rather a gut problem. I then told her about Professor Hunter and his revelation that the idea of 'wear and tear' being a primary cause was now considered archaic (see chapter 27).

"What do you mean ... are you saying my doctor's wrong?"

"Look," I said, "advances made in medical research don't instantly gain acceptance. In 2011 opinions regarding arthritis had already started to change in America. It took about five years before these ideas began to take hold in Australia. I was just lucky that I stumbled across doctors who could help me. I found a gastroenterologist who was ahead of the game. Maybe South Africa is lagging behind?"

This stunned Barb. She no longer felt she should immediately sign up to have both hips replaced. Still, I didn't want to create unrealistic expectations, so I added:

"At the end of the day everyone is different, but I do believe my experience may help others. When my book's finished, I'll send you a copy. In the meantime, I can send you a summary of my pain/discomfort records.

You know I think it was just unbelievably fortunate that I found the help I needed. I'm now fit and totally pain free. Ideally I want to age well and so far so good."

Barb was intrigued. She wanted to continue chatting, but I had to tell her,

"It's way past midnight. We can chat again tomorrow. There's lots more I'd like to tell you, but in the meantime I'll email those Pain Records."

ARTHRITIC SENSATIONS IN MY RIGHT LEG (2010 – 2021)

Late 2010: Acute sharp, intense attack in R. hip and leg overnight – short lived (ch.2)

March 2011: Dull ache + fierce "burning" in hip joint (ch.5)

April 2011: Throbbing R. knee + Sick feeling + pegleg gait (ch.5)

May 2011: Major excruciating attack overnight – piercing pain at top of foot in front of ankle (ch.7)

June 2011: Pins and needles tingling in R. leg and foot – numb toes

July 2011: Wave-like sensation of fluid in joint when bending – arthritic pains "stabilised"(ch.8)

August 2011: Residual weak muscles in R. leg strengthened with exercises (ch.9)

September 2011: Stiff tightness around hip – unable to touch toes (ch.9)

October 2011: Discomfort eased post physiotherapy – Tightness relieved post dry-needling (ch.10)

November 2011: Brisk, pain-free walking resumed

December 2011: Asymptomatic – no surgery indicated (ch.16)

January 2012 – April 2014: Barely discernible, residual mild limp

May 2014: Painless, but audible crunch and slip in R. hip (ch.25)

June-July 2014: Referred pain to R. knee (ch.25)

August-October 2014: Gradual decline in mobility (shorter strides + distances)

November 2014: Pronounced grinding discomfort necessitated walking stick use (ch.25)

December 2014: THR

2015 – 2021: Pain free, fit and agile – promising future of ageing well (ch.28)

NOTE: By November 2014 I was no longer free of arthritic discomfort, however there was - no recurrence of those excruciating 2010/11 attacks that had jolted me awake around midnight.

Poor Barb … when we resumed our chat the next day she sounded even more tense.

"Honestly, I can't make sense of your records. You started with intense pain in early 2011. So why were you pain free for almost three years? Also, what caused that crunch you heard? What really gets me is why on earth was your foot sore when you had a problem in your hip? My doctor just told me to expect my pain to steadily get worse and worse."

"Barb, I know. That's exactly why I was so confused to start with. It also explains why the basic 'wear and tear' explanation has been rejected as it doesn't give the patient an adequate understanding of what's going on. I've since learnt that cartilage disintegration doesn't hurt as it doesn't contain nerves. It's the sinews, muscles, tendons, ligaments and nerves outside the joint that cause most of the painful discomfort. At least that's what I found."

"So why the sore foot?"

"Well, this is my understanding. The acute attacks were inflammation flares that impacted on my muscles. Nerves in my leg got pinched by muscle spasms. I think it's the sciatic nerve that can get caught by hip ligaments. It branches and goes all the way down to the ankle."

I should've anticipated Barb's sceptical response:

"That's the first I've heard of inflammation having anything to do with OA."

At that point I suspect it was a case of information overload, so I simply murmured something about OA having previously been incorrectly classified as a noninflammatory condition.

Best leave it at that I thought. What I could have mentioned were the advances in arthritis research which increasingly pointed to inflammatory mediators as a cause. Some doctors in the US even thought that it was no longer appropriate to refer to OA as a degenerative joint disease. I'd even found a website which stated that "if early recognition leads to early prevention, the hip joint can be saved from destroying itself."

Damage inside and outside my hip joint

Instead of reassuring Barb I think I might have unsettled her, which wasn't my intention at all. Fortunately, that evening I was able to share my concerns with Peter. He was as ever a reliable sounding board and well-remembered how I had shied away from surgery when asked: "What about the pain?"

Immediately he reminded me that we'd decided to use the Oxford Hip Score as a form of objective measure to help me decide whether a THR was needed. This was because my pain trajectory hadn't matched the Kellgren-Lawrence grading system which recorded the four stages of cartilage degeneration; viz. 1. Doubtful, 2. Mild/Minimal, 3. Moderate, 4. Severe. Instead of mild to severe, my experience had been the opposite; i.e. severe ... mild ... none! But then of course the large cyst had collapsed in May 2014. Still, why had there been this lack of correlation?

Peter then added: "What happened to that article I found on arthritis pain surrounding a joint, rather than it being only within the joint capsule?"

Thanks to all the records I'd meticulously kept, it didn't take too long before I retrieved what I was looking for. This article together with a couple of extracts I'd printed from *The BMJ* provided answers.

- Luntz, S.,2012: *"Arthritis Pain is outside the Joints".* Australasian Science, 9:July/August.

"2014 BMJ article: As articular cartilage is aneural it is not a tissue from which pain originates. Sources of pain are – ligament strain, muscle spasm, pinched nerves – secondary to [transient toxic synovitis], an inflammatory response.

BMJ note: In OA the severity and progression of symptoms correlate poorly with the severity and progression of structural damage shown on x-rays. Severity of radiographic change may be a poor predictor of OA pain. Joint loading/weight can be a significant predictor [of pain progressing]."

Professor Hunter had warned in his ABC interview that "joint flexion under load increased the risk of damage." In May 2014 I'd overconfidently flexed my hip joint and placed my full weight on it while yanking on a pair of jeans. This foolish act had caused the cyst to collapse and hastened the end stage. Within six months I couldn't manage without a walking stick. Eventually in December 2014 the discomfort caused by bone grinding on bone had become disabling; no cartilage was left as a cushion between ball and socket.

But what about the severest pain in 2011 that wasn't within my hip joint? By far the worst piercing pain had occurred in the middle of the night. The memory of me scrunched up into a foetal position with my thumbs firmly pressed into the top of my ankle remains crystal clear. Curiously, it was located at the top of my foot in front of my ankle and as I'd explained to Barb, it was caused by inflamed muscles pinching a nerve. Twice I'd experienced such excruciating night-time pain which had rudely awoken me from a deep slumber. Was there an explanation for those midnight attacks? Could changes in blood flow that occur during sleep have provided an opportunity for toxins to accumulate? This is something medical researchers can't yet answer.

The article by Luntz also didn't explain all the sensations that I believe were the result of 'transient toxic synovitis'. Yes, there certainly were inflamed muscles, but also inflamed synovium which caused a fierce burning together with a wave-like sensation of fluid in my joint when I tried bending to spontaneously pluck unsightly weeds. According to the Merck Manual when "the synovium becomes inflamed [it] produces synovial fluid with less viscosity and greater volume."

Thanks to luck and determination this myriad array of symptoms was successfully treated by the functional medicine doctor, a talented physiotherapist and an infectious disease specialist. Eventually the grinding of bone on bone that followed three years later required the skills of a surgeon.

To my mind my case history of the pain and discomfort that I experienced points to transient toxic synovitis and accompanying inflammation as the initiating factor which resulted in the erosion of the cartilage in my right hip. 'Wear and tear' of cartilage was not painful; my pain came from inflammation.

OA, RA, Ankylosing Spondylitis and possibly subclinical septic arthritis

Fate had intervened when I serendipitously heard the ABC interview explaining the shifting sands within the body of medical knowledge about arthritis (see chapter 27). It turned out that I was right to have questioned the 2011 diagnosis I'd been given; viz.

"You have osteoarthritis. It's a chronic and degenerative condition caused by wear and tear."

By 2017, thanks to Professor Hunter, the startling about turn that had occurred in medical understanding was clarified. He and Dr Norman Swan had jokingly talked about their medical training in the 1980s and how they'd been taught theories that were now considered "prehistoric ... belonging to the Jurassic period."

Every aspect of those dated theories had recently been overturned; viz.

'wear and tear', degenerative with age, noninflammatory.

Good studies had shown these ideas were simply incorrect. Even the actual name of the disease (osteoarthritis) was being questioned and some doctors in the US were predicting that eventually the nebulous tag 'idiopathic' would be discarded. It was possible that the term OA could become obsolete.

Clearly my erosive arthritis was unlikely to be a phenomenon with no initiating factor. With the rejection of the 'wear and tear' idea (cartilage starting to spontaneously crumble with age), came the need for me to find an alternative, more plausible explanation. My condition wasn't a 'wear and tear' problem, but rather according to Dr Golledge, I had a very mild autoimmune disorder (see chapter 27).

Fortunately, I'd learnt from the functional medicine doctor that our immune system can be strengthened with an immune modulator like vitamin D3. He'd even published a paper on the topic. Research scientists were investigating the associations between vitamin D deficiency and "so-called autoimmune diseases" like rheumatoid arthritis.

It then dawned on me that I'd been barking up the wrong tree as it were. If I was to understand and take control of my arthritic condition I needed to inform myself about RA not OA. To me the notion that I'd had a brief brush with RA and Ankylosing Spondylitis in 1997 was plausible. It seemed reasonable to deduce that I'd experienced a repeat occurrence in 2011. The acute, excruciating attack around midnight in May 2011 was a painful inflammation flare. RA of course is an inflammatory disease with ongoing flares. According to Phelps it can sometimes start in a single joint and then will spread to other joints. I now felt sure that this was what happened to me, with an inflammation flare in my right hip followed by throbbing in my right knee. The difference being that the course of my disease was halted. The functional medicine doctor successfully stabilised my arthritis. Instead of having to suffer persistent chronic synovitis, what I suffered was transient; but it was toxic nevertheless. The right hip cartilage matrix was irreparably damaged and scarred by features such as a 'wind-sock shaped paralabral cyst'.

The challenge that faced me was to keep my arthritis at bay. For the first time in eight years I again referred to the self-help guide by Jenner, but this time I turned to the section that discussed RA. Both he and Jenkins mentioned mysterious periods of remission. What I didn't want was to deal with unpredictability. I hoped for more certainty; more control. Maybe the answer lay in identifying a likely trigger? Both UK authors mentioned infection as a possibility, but although research was ongoing as yet no conclusive answers had been found.

Admittedly I couldn't conclude with absolute certainty that my cartilage erosion had been initiated by subclinical septic arthritis and/or transient toxic synovitis. What I could claim though was that since 2012 my preventative program seemed to be working. By maintaining a healthy immune system, I intended to continue to keep a lid on infective agents that could spark episodes of transient toxic synovitis. My aim was to receive positive feedback from my surgeon in 2021 as I wanted my arthritis story to end on a high note.

Conclusion

As my eventful decade began to draw to a close, my kind and wise advisor remained true to his word. To further encourage me to complete my story, Dr Hira Singh wrote part of the foreword that he'd promised:

"Antigenic material from biological pathogens triggers the formation of antigen-antibody complexes resulting in inflammation – now recognized as the key pathway leading to dysfunction in multiple organ systems in the body."

Wandering up the shady lane on my return home I started to process this medical and for me rather technical, explanation. A lot had been clarified, but a major question remained. What was the underlying cause - the source of these toxic inflammatory mediators?

I felt the end of my investigative journey was tantalizingly close, but a big question remained. If my treatment was to be reliably effective I needed to confirm what the likely root cause of my 'infective problem' had been.

Chapter 29 INFLAMMATORY MEDIATORS (2019)

The diagnosis of OA in 2011 had caused me to veer off course with my investigations. Even though I'd instinctively reasoned that the 'wear and tear' explanation didn't make sense, it took many years before I began to consider the possibility that my form of arthritis was possibly more closely aligned with RA.

The first book on arthritis that I'd borrowed from the Nedlands library had been written by an RA patient (see chapter 9). Jenkins had suffered from RA for more than thirty years and had had the misfortune of not being diagnosed for ten years. At the time this made me wonder whether subclinical conditions could be particularly challenging to diagnose. However, the sections in her book that interested me were her "personal scenarios" where she described her throbbing wrists which she'd tucked under a pillow at night. I could relate to her description of an inflammation flare, just as I did to the statement in Phelps's text: "RA may present with an acute onset of pain, with peak intensity reached within hours." There's no doubt this was what had jolted me awake in May 2011 (see chapter 7), but what really bothered me was that Phelps went on to say that a presentation of RA could start "as acute monoarthritis, before spreading to other joints." By 2019 I should've felt totally confident that I'd got a firm handle on my arthritis, however I couldn't be certain. Some friends and acquaintances around my age had also had joints replaced. Not all enjoyed the same successful results and just as Phelps mentioned, their arthritis had progressed to other joints.

At that point I recalled a quote from Gandi, made within the context of widespread poverty:

"Look for the cause – don't just treat the symptoms. Treat the underlying cause."

This quote resonated with me, but as a solution to my arthritis.

Arthritis-infection link

Given the experience of friends I felt uneasy and returned to look for information in the texts lining the 'arthritis shelf' in my study. Again, I consulted Phelps's chapter on joints and connective tissues and found further advice for health practitioners when diagnosing monoarthritis:

"Infection should be suspected [with acute onset presentation]. Infectious monoarthritis is an important diagnosis to make early, as joint damage can occur if untreated."

The penny dropped! This explained why the doctor online in the USA had been so prompt with his diagnosis once I'd listed my symptoms (see chapter 2).

According to Jenkins, research was ongoing into whether there was an association between RA and infection. This got me wondering what glimmerings of light might have been uncovered since she published her book in 2011. Surely the Arthritis Foundation who'd encouraged me to take control of my condition would be aware of recent findings. On the spur of the moment, I decided to take the quick drive down to the centre.

It was good that I arrived during a lull in activities, so an assistant in the bookshop had time to chat. We talked a bit about antibiotics and I mentioned how effective macrodantin had been in relieving the throbbing in my right leg (see chapter 2). Yet at the time it was just pure luck that I'd had a urine infection at the time that needed treatment. To my surprise she told me that actually quite a few doctors were now using antibiotics with their RA patients. This was exciting news, so of course I asked if she had any material on these latest treatments. I then learnt that lots of scientific papers had been published on the topic, but no she didn't have anything to give me. However, after a moment's thought she went over to a shelf and pulled out a book.

"You know I think you'd find this interesting. It covers past and current research efforts to establish a connection between RA and infections."

- Brownstein, D., 2001: *Overcoming arthritis*, Medical Alternatives Press, Michigan, USA.

I bought the book and from the very first page I was captivated. There were several complimentary forewords written by highly qualified health practitioners. A "new medical breakthrough" was mentioned, and the title of the chapter that followed the introduction was: The Arthritis-Infection Connection.

Treatment based on clinical observation

My mind was reeling. I knew from the arthritis research website that the "transient toxic synovitis" which had been picked up on my MRI in June 2011 was a damaging "pathological state". However, this condition "could be completely resolved with treatment." It was thanks to serendipity; pure luck that I'd stumbled across exactly the right treatment; just what was needed to stop the infectious arthritis in its tracks before any more damage was done. It made me shudder slightly to realise that I'd probably narrowly escaped the fate that had befallen Jane Fonda who uncomplainingly admitted that her "body hurt almost all the time" (see chapter 26).

Soon afterwards I found myself back in Dr Singh's surgery ever hopeful that he could further enlighten me. Brownstein's book had been a revelation and as I spoke about it my GP simply gave a satisfied shrug and nodded, saying:

"I know I've been successfully treating arthritis for years."

He must've seen that I was dumbfounded, after all how could this be? So he added,

"You see there's often some professional jealousy between doctors."

"But why could a doctor in the USA diagnose my 'cyst' problem and recommend treatment; yet at first here I was left floundering? If it wasn't for Dr Brennan I wouldn't have found you!"

"Well you see modern medicine is evidence based. I believe in my treatment because I know from many years of experience that it works, but my clinical observations aren't considered statistically significant."

"But you could publish a paper!" I said with exasperation.

"I wouldn't waste my time," he said.

With this I was reminded of Dr Barry Marshall's experience and how difficult it was to get successful therapies recognised (see chapter 25). Clear cut evidence is required.

RA treatment lost & found

It upset me to think advances in effective arthritis treatment could be so achingly slow. I was stunned to learn as I read Brownstein's chapter, that "it has been known for over one hundred years that mycoplasma organisms are able to cause arthritis symptoms." However, right at the start of his book he made it clear that "in conventional medicine there was no consensus on what causes arthritis." But then his work had been published in 2001. Ten years later when Phelps's tome was released, there'd at last been a shift in the medical understanding of arthritis. It was reassuring to find that common causes of RA listed under 'aetiology' were: genetic, microbial (mycobacterial/bacterial), immunological factors and autoimmune disease.

What I'd uncovered fascinated me. It was extraordinary that doctors had first suspected many types of arthritis could be some form of 'infective problem' as far back as the late 1800s. This made me wonder whether some sort of rivalry between medical researchers was hindering advancement. I recalled the shenanigans that were described in Shilts's book on the AIDS epidemic (see chapter 21). Mischief had occurred between the French and the Americans in the race to isolate a culprit.

Sure enough, the pioneering achievements of Dr McPherson Brown on antibiotic treatment for RA had not received the recognition they deserved. This rheumatologist pursued his line of research into an "unorthodox treatment" for RA throughout his career. What he considered to be curative treatment failed to attract attention as his work was completely overshadowed by a new wonder drug called cortisone. Unfortunately for the patients the relief cortisone brought came at a price. After years of regular injections many RA patients landed up with osteoporosis. Sometimes research efforts can be derailed by the bright lights of seemingly miraculous treatments, only to find years later that apparent success came at the cost of serious long-term side effects.

Even I'd had a narrow escape. To this day I can recall begging a specialist to,

"Just pump me full of cortisone and I'll be fine."

He'd looked me straight in the eye and said firmly: "You certainly don't want me to do that to you."

Instead, in 1997 I'd hobbled off to a cobbler who specialised in making shoe inserts for RA patients. Fortunately, those ineffective aids landed up being quickly discarded as shortly afterwards I discovered Campbell's "home cure for arthritis" (see chapter 4).

Possible infective agents/inflammatory mediators:

Campbell's consistent mantra was straightforward and easy to follow:

- Nutrition
- Elimination

- Circulation

My downfall had been a gross lack of elimination of waste left over from digested food. This build-up of waste led to the development of toxic synovitis; a damaging inflammatory process that's not completely understood. However, over the previous decade significant advances in research had been made. In 2011 I'd been utterly puzzled and perplexed when doctors had referred to *'it'*. Initially I'd thought *C.Albicans* mentioned by Jenner in relation to fungal infections, might be the culprit, but Dr Golledge had assured me that this was unlikely. This led me to simply list microbes that were suggested in the texts I'd referred to:

Epstein Barr Virus (Crook's *Yeast connection*)

Klebsiella Bacteria (Weatherby & Gordin's *Arthritis Bible*)

Candida Albicans (Richardson & Warnock's *Fungal Infection*)

Mycobacteria/bacteria (Phelps's *General Practice; the integrative approach*)

Ever curious I decided to return to the Nedlands library. Maybe researchers had pursued the link between bacteria, arthritis and thyroiditis. Sure enough, I was not disappointed as the alert young librarian in no time at all steered me towards a well-stocked shelf of texts covering nutrition. Since my research project began in 2011, an impressive book had been added to the collection.

- Greger, M., 2017: H*ow not to die; discover the foods scientifically proven to prevent and reverse disease,* Pan Macmillan, London, UK.

In Dr Greger's chapter on infections he quoted studies that revealed cases where autoimmune arthritis and autoimmune thyroiditis were diagnosed in almost 50% of patients who'd been victims of a *Yersinia* bacterial infection. However, Dr Brownstein's list of agents that caused "infectious arthritis" was much longer, but the lead contender for this not particularly salubrious aetiological arthritis role appeared to be a bacterium called mycoplasma.

I felt that these findings provided yet more evidence that my health issues could well have been the result of an 'infective problem'.

Having finally reached this point in my investigative story gave me a huge sense of achievement. At last, I could suggest that a bacterium was a likely causative agent for my arthritis and thyroiditis. I'd come a long way since late 2011 when I'd sat down and compiled a list of risk factors that were possibly underlying a condition that had been crippling (see chapter 12). Towards the end of that year I'd already started to speculate whether "bacteria were causing the inflammations in arthritic conditions such as RA and ankylosing spondylitis."

My sense of accomplishment was strengthened by the realisation that many of the risk factors I'd compiled were now recognised by mainstream medicine.

The 'infection versus trauma' debate

Come August 2019, I eagerly packed for a trip to Tassie with a group of friends. It was a planned ten-year reunion. The three couples arranged to fly into Hobart where we met up in a grand old Sandy Bay mansion that had been converted into B & B apartments.

Each of the seven days together were carefully planned, and day one started with a boat trip up the River Derwent to the extraordinary MONA Gallery. Of course there was a lot of chatting; so much to catch up on after such a long time. While the boys discussed sport and politics, the girls brought each other up to date as to what we'd been doing now our children were married and off our hands.

Kate had been a maths teacher and was now a scientist, while Bev had returned to nursing part-time. When asked what I'd been up to I briefly described my arthritis project which had turned into a ten-year study of a sample of one. I hastily added that I wouldn't have embarked on such a lengthy project if it wasn't for the encouragement of my doctors and Peter's unwavering support.

"But what prompted this study?" Kate asked.

"Well ... I just couldn't accept my initial diagnosis and prognosis."

Given what I'd recently discovered I added that the old 'wear and tear' theory for OA had been discarded and I believed the causative factor for my arthritis had been an 'infective problem'. To my astonishment this sparked a heated debate. Bev loudly and firmly asserted that "No, cartilage degeneration is caused by trauma!" With that, Kate thrust forward her hand and showed us her crooked arthritic fingers that I'd not previously noticed. Firmly shaking her head she told me that my explanation sounded more plausible. At least Kate, with her recent scientific training, was prepared to be open minded, so I went on to elaborate about Dr McPherson Brown's antibiotic therapy. Like me Kate was fascinated, but then added: "I guess doctors still need to determine just which antibiotics are the most effective." I nodded and added that in my view antibiotic therapy formed the initial stage of a comprehensive holistic treatment program. Such a program needed to be multidisciplinary, involving allied professions; for example nutritionists and physiotherapists. It was this sort of program that I'd found enormously beneficial.

Conclusion:

As 2019 drew to a close I felt encouraged as I'd begun to find support for my belief in antibiotic therapy and also for My Theoretical Concept (see Figure 8). At the start of 2011 my ideas had been considered controversial by mainstream medicine and were simply rejected (see chapter 3). However, the ABC radio interview that I'd listened to in 2017 with Professor Hunter had marked a turning point in my investigative journey. It was a relief to hear him talk plainly and openly to Dr Norman Swan about arthritis (see chapter 27). There were no ifs, buts, or maybes. Instead in a matter-of-fact manner he debunked existing 'wear and tear', degenerative and non-inflammatory theories regarding OA.

What my intuition had told me right from the start with the acute, painful onset, was validated. That excruciating attack and the throbbing that ensued were caused by an 'infective problem', which was why I'd responded quickly to the antibiotic macrodantin. Today many specialists now recognise that infectious microbes cause certain forms of arthritis. I'd been right to question the dismal diagnosis and prognosis that I'd been given (see chapter 3). With Professor Hunter's validation came the realisation that a key feature of My Theoretical Concept (see Figure 8) had been verified; viz.

- Inflammation and/or infection (the result at the bottom of my flowchart)

Greatly encouraged I started to hope that the central piece of My Concept might also gain some recognition; viz.

- My damaged gut.

Chapter 30 AN OVERLOOKED RISK FACTOR (2020)

In 2020 I continued to enjoy good health and wonder-of-wonders I remained pain free. This apparently mystified the medical profession as my GP had commented that I was "confounding doctors." But instinctively I knew why I'd fully recovered and remained fit and well. In large part it was thanks to the book by Dr Campbell that I'd found in the depths of the Notre Dame University library in 1997. His three-step advice to healing primarily emphasised "elimination", and he described arthritis as a "toxic condition". When I'd discussed his methods with Dr Singh, he'd agreed but added that sadly this helpful information had probably been dismissed by modern medicine. Indeed, he was right as I'd been told early on in 2011 that it was "rubbish" (see chapter 3).

The conservative, mainstream physician whom I'd encountered at the beginning of this arthritis story had stubbornly refused to accept my ideas. I'd been patronisingly told that an infection couldn't have moved from my bowel to my hip. Instead of arguing, I'd simply remembered the American doctor's advice and decided to further investigate such a possibility. The next text that I consulted following Campbell's was a lengthy volume by Dr Crook. It was filled with useful information, successful case studies, simple flow charts and diagrams. Illustrations that particularly intrigued me were of *Candida albicans,* a noxious microbe that was capable, according to Richardson and Warnock, of "translocating" across the epithelial barrier of my gut (see chapter 21). Dr Crook described it as a Dr Jekyll and Mr

Hyde organism that could morph. Initially I had trouble visualizing the antics of such a pesky critter, so I decided to create illustrations of my own based on images on medical websites (see Figure 9).

As with Campbell I'd found Dr Crook's theories convincing, and I again became engrossed in what he had to say, particularly regarding the colon.

Constipation

As described in chapter 13 I'd endured severe, chronic constipation for most of my life and consequently I'd damaged my bowel. I've also mentioned that physically I'm very much a clone of my mother, yet she remained fit and active all her life and to my knowledge neither she nor her three siblings (two sisters and a brother) had to have joints replaced. Why had I been afflicted? Was there something I should've paid attention to and corrected? Indeed ... there was.

My mother had known that I had a tendency to become constipated as a little girl . She herself had occasionally had such a problem, which was why an old-fashioned remedy had always been available in the medicine cabinet; viz. Phillip's Milk of Magnesia. Unfortunately, by the time I started school our new family physician's attitude regarding regular BMs was very laid back. The young doctor relayed to my mother what he'd been taught at medical school, which was:

"Forget about your child's bowel movements. It makes no difference whether she has a bowel movement twice a day or once a week. So-called toxins from the colon are a myth."

These days I've come to understand how the medical pendulum can swing. There'd been the move from one medication to another; e.g. cortisone rather than antibiotic therapy. A similar phenomenon had also occurred regarding the medical profession's attitude towards bowel movements. As Campbell and Crook had belonged to my mother's generation their attitude was that daily elimination of toxic waste was vital. By the time I'd turned five, most doctors no longer paid any attention to the regularity of bowel movements.

Unfortunately for me I was left to cope as best I could, and my gut continued to limp along with its pathetic pellet-like droppings for more than 50 years. It's not surprising that by the time I reached 58 years of age in 2011, things had begun to go seriously awry with a myriad of ailments appearing, ranging from skin issues to a peg-leg gait. My acute arthritis attack that year had been a wake-up call. Fortunately, I'd found old-school medical texts that drew my attention to my feeble bowel habits. This was just as well, as the first doctors I sought help from paid absolutely no heed as to whether I was eliminating waste or not. It was thanks to Campbell's book that I'd requested a colonoscopy. This had marked a turning point (see chapter 5).

The request for a colonoscopy in 2011 had led me to meet Dr Brennan, the Irish gastroenterologist. After the procedure he'd chatted to me about my constipation and my recently diagnosed arthritis. He'd alerted me to the importance of maintaining a healthy immune function and suggested I see Dr Singh as he'd be able to provide me with the advice I needed. It had taken four months before I managed to get an appointment with this doctor who was in high demand. In the interim I'd been lucky enough to obtain just the help I needed at the time from a functional medicine doctor. He'd immediately recognised that I had a gut health problem, in particular chronic constipation. From the information he gave me I was led to believe that he also suspected a link - possibly a root cause - between my gut health and my arthritis.

The term 'idiopathic' (cause unknown) is still used by some doctors in relation to arthritis, but I maintain that in my case the underlying cause of my arthritis was effectively treated by the functional medicine doctor. What I consider to be a fundamental risk factor for my form of arthritis was recognised and promptly addressed. Yet it continues to astonish me that despite years of positive clinical observations the treatments offered by the functional medicine doctor are still not more widely acknowledged by conventional medicine.

The Hunter-Gatherer Diet linked to good health and less disease

Successful treatment that fails to achieve recognition is not an uncommon theme in medicine. A particularly high-profile example is that of Dr Barry Marshall which I related in chapter 25. From my perspective both doctors Campbell and Crook were pioneers in the area of toxic inflammatory conditions that were related to gut health. Their treatments zeroed in on a fresh wholefood fibre-rich diet. Processed foods were to be avoided.

Crook discussed how his interest in the hunter-gatherer diet had been piqued by the work of a famous English physician; a Dr Denis Burkitt. This doctor studied the diets of Africans for 25 years and found a significant correlation between health problems and diet. The Africans who'd adopted a western diet weren't as healthy as the more primitive tribes.

A small tribe of true hunter-gatherers - the Hadzas - still lives on the edge of the Serengeti in Tanzania and at present research is ongoing into links between their health, lifestyle and diet. Unsurprisingly their gut health is excellent as their native diet with lots of fruits and fibre-rich tubers ensures regularity – two to four BMs per day. This high-fibre diet which is low in processed sugars and contains phytochemicals, is thought to contribute to their good health and well-being. Chronic illnesses such as diabetes, colon cancer, arthritis and autoimmune diseases barely exist. Obesity is unheard of as these people remain slim and active.

Crook went on to discuss how he followed research results in medical journals in the 1980s that confirmed Burkitt's observations. He also noted that apparently "toxins of various sorts are absorbed from the intestinal tract of people whose diets are low in fibre, but high in fat, sugar and protein." He then quoted a fellow physician stating that:

"When a person's colon is loaded with impacted faecal material, *C.Albicans* [and other hostile microbes] thrive."

These research findings were made more than thirty years ago. Crook, who came from a line of medical practitioners, ended his discussion on a confident note stating that:

"There's growing scientific evidence from many sources that my father and grandfather may have known something [about the importance of gut health] back in the 1920s."

Yet 100 years later, I found these ideas still weren't widely recognised by mainstream medicine. It continues to frustrate me that clear cut research evidence is required for successful basic therapies (antibiotic therapy) and interventions (gut treatment) to be generally adopted.

Permeability of intestines officially recognised

In October 2011, thanks to the functional medicine doctor, I'd decided to take charge of my health; to steer my own course. So I'd drawn up my own guidelines which began with two logical steps (see chapter 12):

Step 1: Identify possible underlying causes and/or trigger factors.

Step 2: Address each factor and determine a solution.

Unfortunately, many came to regard my ideas as fanciful notions; evidence that I was unhinged. It was a heavy price to pay for having an enquiring mind.

Nevertheless, it continues to irk me that a basic concept that could well be a root cause for many forms of arthritis fails to be accepted by mainstream medicine; viz. chronic constipation damaging one's bowel and causing intestinal permeability.

Peter, however, remained steadfast in his support, as did Dr Singh. They encouraged me to persevere with my investigative story into what might explain my arthritic attacks. I still hoped to substantiate My Concept (my theoretical understanding) of the underlying causes (see Figure 8).

When I'd searched the web for more information about this phenomenon of toxins from the colon causing inflammation, I'd found several naturopathic websites describing the "Leaky Gut Syndrome" in detail. Dr Singh had assured me this information was correct and had added that the gut strongly influences our immune function as our intestines house over two-thirds of our immune cells. Even though many doctors continued to dismiss this syndrome that naturopaths and functional medicine doctors were successfully treating, peer reviewed articles had begun to appear in medical journals (2018-20) which confirmed that gut permeability was real.

In the midst of this ongoing controversy that existed between mainstream and alternative medicine, Peter managed to find a book that resolved the debate; that recognised a gut condition now known as "intestinal permeability". To my utter delight, in July 2020, Peter presented me with this perfect birthday gift.

- Bird, T. and others, 2018: *The CSIRO Healthy Gut Diet*, Macmillan Publishers, Sydney, Australia.

This was no ordinary recipe book. In large part it was scientific, based on 20 years or more of research, and provided medical advice regarding gut related health issues. The blurb on the flyleaf captured my attention:

"In recent years, we've come to realise that a healthy gut is pivotal to a healthy metabolism, a healthy brain and a healthy immune system."

So by 2020 there'd been an astonishingly rapid increase in the number of scientific studies worldwide in the field of gut health. But Australia's CSIRO was at the forefront of this research which led to the discovery of a key dietary ingredient that reinforced the epithelial gut barrier. Like the forerunners, Campbell and Crook, a fresh whole-food diet high in fibre was stressed, but they'd taken this advice a step further. Different types of fibre were specified and one in particular was highlighted:

"Resistant starch is the real gold – it promotes gut-wall integrity, healthy digestion and optimal immune function."

Scientists had discovered that this type of starch was fermented by the microbiota in our large intestine. This set a process in motion which nourished our gut barrier and gut mucosa; i.e.

1. enzymes fermented the resistant starch
2. short-chain fatty acids were produced – notably butyrate
3. a fuel (butyrate) was provided for the epithelial cells of the large bowel

This gave me specific dietary advice to help restore and maintain a strong and healthy bowel wall. Of course, that wasn't the only health benefit. Several others were discussed ranging from preventing constipation to reducing the risk of bowel cancer.

Once I knew for certain that the measures I'd taken from late 2011 onwards should've promoted my gut wall integrity, I became curious as to what changes, if any, might have occurred in the wall of my damaged right colon (see chapters 13 & 24, and Figure 4). Could it have healed itself? I wondered if those pouches in my large bowel might have at least shrunk, if not withered into flat sacks like skin tags.

The inner skin's ability to repair

Before I got too carried away with these ideas of gut wall repair, I thought I'd have a quick chat with a GP. Dr Singh was away but his partner, whom I'd met on previous occasions, was open to such possibilities but agreed that at best I might be left with fragments of those diverticula. So many years of chronic constipation had probably scarred my bowel wall. But still he readily gave me a referral to see Dr Brennan and I was lucky to get an appointment that November.

Ever curious and with time on my hands before I'd again get to see the gut specialist, I returned to my study to see if I could unearth more information about damaged bowel walls and the possibilities of repair. Doidge's book had taught me in early 2012 that the liver was one organ that could completely regenerate. I then found in his chapter on "Rejuvenation" that "several [other] parts of the human body are able to regenerate after an injury". Our outer skin was one of those parts, but so too was our inner skin.

This clarified why the CSIRO text described our gut like a "tube lined by a continuation of our skin called the epithelium." From previous readings I'd learnt that our gut barrier consists of a layer of these epithelial cells which line our intestines. It's this crucial mucosal barrier that controls "the paracellular pathway (a route for 'translocation' of molecules between cells)". Richardson and Warnock had also described this 'translocation' of microbes across the bowel wall into the bloodstream.

As I had trouble visualising these "paracellular pathways" I turned to a scientific website of medical images to see what I could find. Sure enough, there were several freely available diagrams illustrating this 'translocation' process. From this information I created an image of the two pathways that toxic molecules could use to cross the gut's epithelium: the transcellular pathway and the paracellular pathway (see Figure 13). These illustrations reinforced My Concept that a damaged bowel could lead to an increase in the translocation of toxins as "paracellular pathways are regulated by intact tight junctions." It seemed obvious that those "tight junctions" would've been compromised by the pressure and stretching that came with faecal impaction.

To add to the evidence of gut permeability I discovered more about the nature of *bacterial mycoplasmas;* the lead aetiological agents for RA that Dr McPherson Brown had isolated (see chapter 29). These pesky critters are even more devious than *C. albicans*. It made me slightly shudder to learn that such minuscule bacteria are "capable of shedding their cell walls, allowing their essential parts to persist in the form of a gel (plasma), thus giving the organism a better chance of hiding from the host's defences." In this infinitesimal form they could take advantage of microscopic slipways between epithelial cells where tight junctions had been damaged.

Apparently, scientists have also found that some germs associated with inflammatory arthritis are surrounded by smaller organisms that look like jellyfish; an 'L-form' that bacteria can adopt. This made me recall my gut's response to treatments in 2011 and the glossy blobs that had been expelled. Oddly enough I'd used the word 'jellyfish' to describe them (see chapter 24). It was an interesting speculation but nevertheless intriguing. Maybe I'd actually sighted those troublesome microbes.

All this evidence convinced me that the inflammation and throbbing I'd experienced in my right leg was the result of an increase in the translocation of toxic microbes across my gut barrier. As the throbbing had ceased in 2011 with antibiotic therapy and my leg had remained free of such discomfort for almost ten years, I felt confident that there was the possibility my gut had indeed healed. Surely my inner skin had repaired itself by growing new cells.

By returning to talk to the gently spoken Irish gastroenterologist I hoped to bring my story to a close. But would I be able to end my ten-year study on a triumphant note?

November 2020: Surprising results from a GI review

With COVID-19 upsets and lockdowns, my chances of getting an appointment before the end of the year had been slim. But, fortunately on a Monday morning in early November I'd made the brief walk through an unbelievably heavy downpour, back to the Hollywood specialist centre.

By the time I arrived my shoes were sodden and my coat completely soaked. Before sitting down in the gastro specialist's neat office, I peeled off my new, navy raincoat which made for a friendly opening to our discussion; a bit of banter about the need for such coats in Ireland, but rarely in Perth, Western Australia.

Seven years had passed since I'd last sat in that room, yet it felt like yesterday. The memories flooded back. For me it was easy. The recollections were still very clear. Unsurprisingly, Dr Brennan needed to refer to his records; the colonoscopy reports from 2011 and 2013.

What I'd long suspected was confirmed. In 2011 damage had been noted in my right colon. Diverticula, or pouches were detected. Probably the result of decades of severe constipation. Yet the colonoscopy report in 2013 revealed that my gastro-intestinal tract was "entirely normal".

Like Dr Golledge, Dr Brennan had said "we don't really know why some patients get better", however he had a close friend who focussed on research into the GI microbiome. Apparently impressive research findings were steadily accumulating, much like snow on a mountain top. He forecast that an avalanche of information was coming.

Dr Brennan then ordered a CRP assay blood test; an inflammation marker. For me it was the cherry on the top, as it indicated an absence of inflammation caused by a bacterial infection.

This good news renewed my enthusiasm. At last I could confidently proceed and complete my story without the fear of being ridiculed. Then by making his records available to me - by saying "anyone can read what I write" - Dr Brennan gave me something precious ... encouragement.

December 2020: Conclusion

My ongoing treatment plan - which included the CSIRO dietary guidelines - had continued to work.

Arthritic attacks hadn't come back to haunt me. I remained fit and well and able to enjoy brisk walks down to the banks of the Swan to spot pelicans, black swans, and even dolphins. Occasionally I would burst into a run just for the thrill of it.

Dr Hira Singh was vindicated. In 2011 he'd confidently predicted "You will get your miracle".

EPILOGUE (2021)

My ten-year study of a sample of one came to an end in May 2021. That excruciating midnight attack that had left me weeping many years ago, had become a dim and distant memory (see chapter 7). As I'd said to Dr Brennan at my November 2020 appointment, I felt 100% well, as did my sister who also took good care of her health and maintained fitness. I admired the way she began each day with an ocean swim. But then quite out of the blue, we received terribly shocking news from Melbourne. She'd had an horrific accident which could've killed her.

Osteoporosis

In September 2021 I heard my mobile ping. A message had come in from my sister Susan. She'd sent me a beautiful picture of a cherry tree in full bloom. How lovely I thought ... the first signs of spring. How wrong I was. Her message alarmed me as she'd taken the photo from her hospital bed where she was racked with pain and immobile. She was waiting to be wheeled to the theatre for major surgery needed to piece together the splintered bones in her knee and lower leg. Immediately I rang her and only just in time. As briefly as she could she explained what had happened and assured me that she was about to receive the very best of surgical care. The following day I learnt more about how she'd fallen and why a five-hour operation had been required.

She and Martin had been taking a refreshing, early morning stroll along Sorrento beach when they'd reached a wooden groyne crossing their path. Martin went ahead and dropped down over the low barrier; with that Susan had unhesitatingly followed. At that moment her leg gave way beneath her to the sound of a sharp crack. All the pleasures of their solitary walk evaporated as she lay there in agony. But Martin, ever cool, calm and collected had immediately called an ambulance. Within the shortest possible time she'd been ferried to the best hospital on the Mornington Peninsula.

As Susan told me the story she sounded fiercely determined, saying

"Mary Anne don't worry I'm going to get the help of physiotherapists. Just like you I'm going to rehabilitate myself ... I'll be walking by Christmas!"

Determination must run in the family, but in my sister's case her recovery post-surgery was not going to be a walk in the park as mine had been. Her ailment was severe osteoporosis; it was life threatening, unlike my OA. Fortunately, an exceptional surgeon was on hand who'd been able to use bone donated from America, as grafting was needed to piece together her shattered tibia. Her situation was so serious, amputation would have been considered had such exceptional medical expertise not been on hand.

Alarm bells began ringing as I recalled an image in Jenner's text depicting the porous, brittle nature of osteoporosis. It was thanks to this book that I'd asked Dr Golledge in 2012 for a referral to get a Bone Mineral Density (BMD) test done. Fortunately, that test when I was 58 years of age, was a warning that I had osteopenia; I needed to take measures to stop osteoporosis from developing. Ever diligent I'd added Ostelin to my collection of brekkie supplements.

Now in November 2021 the question was whether the Ostelin and extra vitamin D3 that I'd been taking for ten years had successfully staved off a debilitating bone disease. Mercifully Dr Singh's broad smile instantly reassured me when I went to see him, having completed another BMD test.

"Your bone density is above the mean for your age and you're not shrinking. You don't have osteoporosis."

Thanks to my supplements I was still standing tall and erect and it wasn't just Ostelin and vitamin D3 that I'd been taking. I'd also added vitamin K2. This wonder vitamin had oddly enough been brought to my attention by the COVID pandemic as I'd closely been following on YouTube the rise in cases across the globe. Along with the alarming statistics a number of impressive physicians had taken it upon themselves to offer advice based on up to the minute research. By 2021 research was showing how vitamin K2 was also beneficial as it helped bind calcium to our bones.

One morning as I watched the latest COVID update on the UK situation, I'd also learnt about Ireland handing out bottles of vitamin D3 when people turned up for their COVID jabs. It had finally been clinically proven that Vitamin D3 was an effective immune modulator; something the functional medicine doctor had known when he'd prescribed them for me in 2011.

My writing ambition

As my appointment with Dr Singh came to an end, he quietly informed me that he was soon to retire. Of course he knew about my writing project and how I wished to share my good news story with others. At the very least I wanted to complete the first draft manuscript before he disappeared out of my life. So he asked me how far I'd got; perhaps I'd reached a halfway point. Did I think I'd complete the book by the end of the year. To which I replied that maybe if I kept to my demanding schedule, I'd just manage to get it done. I'd like to think he wished to ease the pressure that I'd imposed on myself, as he then firmly said: "I won't be going anywhere until June next year."

On my return home I let Peter know that suddenly I had a deadline to meet and he immediately came up with two constructive suggestions. The first was that he would take charge of all meals: menus, shopping and cooking. The second one was to offer to use his computer to complete diagrams from the sketches I'd drawn. There and then he opened a folder for the figures that I'd completed up to that point and while doing that we made a discovery.

"Do you remember when you thought other arthritis patients like yourself might find an informative pamphlet of flowcharts helpful? Early last year you created one that summarised 'Dysbiosis' and another that explained your theoretical understanding which you referred to as 'My Concept'."

I'd completely forgotten about my attempt to create a pamphlet and I found myself quite surprised by my handiwork. At times I'd thought how many different aspects there were to consider if one was to fully grasp the ramifications of the toxic condition that I'd remedied. Peter was right and with that I added the two additional diagrams that I hoped would summarise my experience and the factors that triggered my arthritis (see Figures 11 and 12).

Objective evidence my arthritis has been stabilised

Besides getting my head around and developing an understanding of the many factors that had caused my form of arthritis, I'd also come to grips with the high standards demanded of researchers. Medical scientists are required to provide absolute, incontrovertible proof of the presence of infective aetiological agents. When the pioneer Dr McPherson Brown isolated mycoplasma lurking in the joints of RA patients it was a minor miracle as technology 100 years ago wasn't that advanced. Even today it's a huge challenge for researchers to isolate mycoplasma given its tricky nature and antics that can render it practically invisible (see chapter 30).

Notwithstanding this, at the end of my ten-year study I'd been able to verify that my bowel was no longer damaged and my skeleton was in good nick. Of course, I also knew that my pain trajectory hadn't matched the steady erosion of cartilage in my right hip. Severe pain had been associated with the acute, excruciating onset associated with toxic synovitis which had responded well to antibiotic therapy and gut treatment (see chapter 28). Unfortunately though, all these positive achievements were subjective and only circumstantial evidence at best. None of this was incontrovertible proof that could substantiate My Concept.

The only other objective evidence that I may be able to provide would be radiographic images. I'd not forgotten how the functional medicine doctor had explained to me in June 2011 that he'd also had the condition. When he added with certainty that he could "stabilise it" I'd simply felt he knew what he was dealing with. He didn't beat about the bush as others had done. Instead, I'd been given printed sheets of useful information that supported the helpful - not harmful – treatment he was offering me (see chapter 8).

In spite of the demands of my punishing writing schedule, Peter encouraged me to go a step further; to obtain clear cut proof from an MRI that my arthritis had been "stabilised" in my right knee – the one that had throbbed. So, towards the end of 2021 I returned to speak to Dr Singh and asked him to request an MRI review of my knee which I offered to pay for. Quite rightly it couldn't be a legitimate medicare claim as I was agile and totally pain free.

Unhesitatingly he agreed and suggested he copy Dr Golledge in on the results. To me this demonstrated an air of optimism which Peter and I responded to. Before the end of the week, I returned to the Medical Diagnostic Imaging Centre that I'd frequented in 2011. Prior to getting the scans done I filled in the required paperwork which requested my email address. To my surprise I learnt that the results - scans and reports - would be sent not just to my GP but also directly to me.

Ten days later a message appeared in my inbox containing a password protected link to my records held by the Imaging Centre. The report was detailed; almost too much information. What delighted me though was to see the word 'stable' used repeatedly. For the purposes of my story all that was needed was the conclusion to make a straightforward comparison between 2011 and 2021.

MRIs OF RIGHT KNEE:

- **20/06/2011:** "Right knee aching at night" - **Small-intermediate depth cartilage thinning** of "the femoral condyle" [i.e. cartilage lining lower end of femur at knee joint].
- **18/11/2021:** "10-year review of right knee" - **STABLE** appearance **of tiny area** of full-thickness **chondral [cartilage] wear** of the femoral condyle.

True to his word, the functional medicine doctor had stopped the throbbing in my knee and stabilised the small amount of cartilage damage that had occurred in 2011.

As I rummaged through all my MRI records, I also came across those that had been taken of my left hip. They'd been part of full pelvic scans which are done as doctors often anticipated patients needing to have both hips replaced eventually. On closer inspection I suddenly realised that they also supported the functional medicine doctor's predictions.

MRIs OF LEFT HIP:

- 3/**10/2014** ... "**LEFT HIP JOINT SPACE PRESERVED** and adequate."
- 12/**12/2014 ... "Relatively mild** degenerative change at the left hip."
- 3/**12/2015 ... "**Compared to 12/12/2014 a little narrowing is noted, [but] **no significant change has occurred**."

The scans of my left hip showed no evidence of ongoing cartilage degeneration ... no 'so-called wear and tear'... but then the left side of my colon had never been damaged.

When I'd shared these results with Peter his enthusiastic response took me by surprise:

"Let's go back to see Dr Witherow. It would be good to ask him for a final review of your left hip seeing as you're about to wrap up your arthritis project."

This time it was with eager anticipation that we returned to the Orthopaedic Centre. Seven years had passed since my THR and Dr Witherow was just the same; as approachable as ever.

"So tell me, why are you here?" he asked.

He then listened intently to me as I explained that I hoped to complete my ten-year arthritis project on a high note. Would he mind if I mentioned his name.

"Look that sounds absolutely fine" was his prompt response. "Now would you like to go straight upstairs and get an X-ray done immediately?"

With that I enthusiastically headed for the lift. In no time at all it was all done and dusted. Dr Witherow beckoned us back into his office where he already had the new images on display. Quickly and professionally he used his pen to point out the relevant features, saying:

"This is what we look for: a decent joint space, absence of cartilage and bone damage, no osteophytes. I can't find fault with your left hip."

Of course, Peter and I were thrilled and even more so when the surgeon who'd looked after me so well added that I didn't need to see him again. I could simply get on with enjoying life.

Conclusion

For me arthritis had been stopped in its tracks.

With satisfaction I recalled the advice Dr Golledge had given me when I'd been uncertain as to how to take care of my health going forward. He'd simply said:

"If what you're doing is working then you're doing the right thing."

Well … what had I done? I'd addressed my Risk Factors and put together a Preventative Regimen which included key vitamins and minerals that had been recommended by the GPs and specialists I'd consulted. This preventative plan remains in place … it continues to work for me.

Yet what gave me the greatest satisfaction was to have successfully unravelled my perplexing arthritis puzzle; to have eventually arrived at a self-explanatory name for my condition:

Right hip cartilage disintegration initiated by corrosive toxic synovitis; a consequence of permeable intestines damaged by chronic constipation (see Figure 14).

But I can't rightly claim I've achieved this all on my own, as there's a reminder on the Harvard University website that:

"INTEGRATIVE MEDICAL PRACTITIONERS HAVE WORKED ON **GUT HEALING** AS AN **INITIAL STEP** TO TREAT CHRONIC DISEASE [SUCH AS ARTHRITIS] FOR DECADES."

POSTSCRIPT

At the end of my appointment with Dr Hira Singh on Monday 11th April 2022, he handed me my annual health report. With immense satisfaction I read:

"Osteoarthritis – in remission."

Dr Jenner's prediction that "in some cases arthritis can even be driven into complete remission," became a reality for me. Ever since 2011 this encouraging statement had been a guiding light. It had filled me with the determination to achieve a goal that I believed was attainable; viz.

To remain active and pain free.

Appendix A FIGURES

12 My Theoretical Concept: an understanding of my arthritis and the gut connection

13 Translocation of microbes through the gut's mucosal barrier

14 Cartilage disintegration initiated by infective toxic synovitis

DATE	SYMPTOMS, AILMENTS, SENSATIONS	MEDICAL OPINION AND STANDARD TREATMENT	MULTI-DISCIPLINARY AND ALTERNATIVE HEALTH CARE	ADDITIONAL INFORMATION SOURCES	MY RESPONSE TO MY ARTHRITIC CONDITION	MY UNDERSTANDING AND/OR APPROACH TO ISSUES	OUTCOMES (pain, flexibility; gait, walking)
Early 1997	Light throbbing in wrists; burning heels	Arthritic-like inflammation	Possibly pre-arthritis	Campbell: *A doctor's proven new home cure for arthritis*	Tension (workplace stress); gut shut-down and severe constipation	Toxic condition	Painful feet, began to hobble
Mid 1997	Sore feet	Possibly ***Rheumatoid Arthritis***; orthotic shoe inserts	Referred to a rheumatologist	Campbell's guidelines	Summarised key points in Campbell's book	Aspirin and foot massages	Fatigued, difficulty walking
Late 1997	Hot 'stickiness' towards top of spine	Possibly ***Ankylosing Spondylitis*** (blood test confirmation); Celebrex	Adopted Campbell's approach: healthy diet, supplements and exercise	Campbell's guidelines	Sense of urgency: took charge of my own health	Supplements: ginseng; ginkgo biloba; multivitamin; cod liver oil	Rapid, full recovery
End 1997	Pain free	No Celebrex; no corticosteroids; no surgery		Campbell's guidelines	Followed Campbell's regime	**Maintenance: good nutrition; daily elimination; exercise/ circulation**	Beginning of 14 years of no symptoms

Figure 1: Arthritic-like inflammation caused by toxic condition in 1997

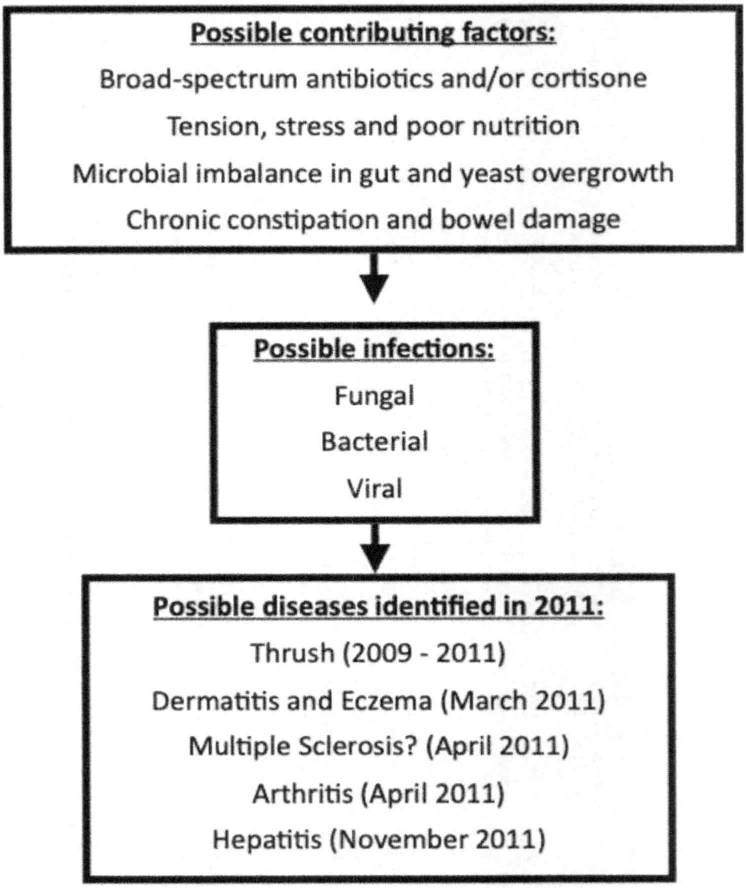

Figure 2: Possible diseases my deficient immune system couldn't keep in check

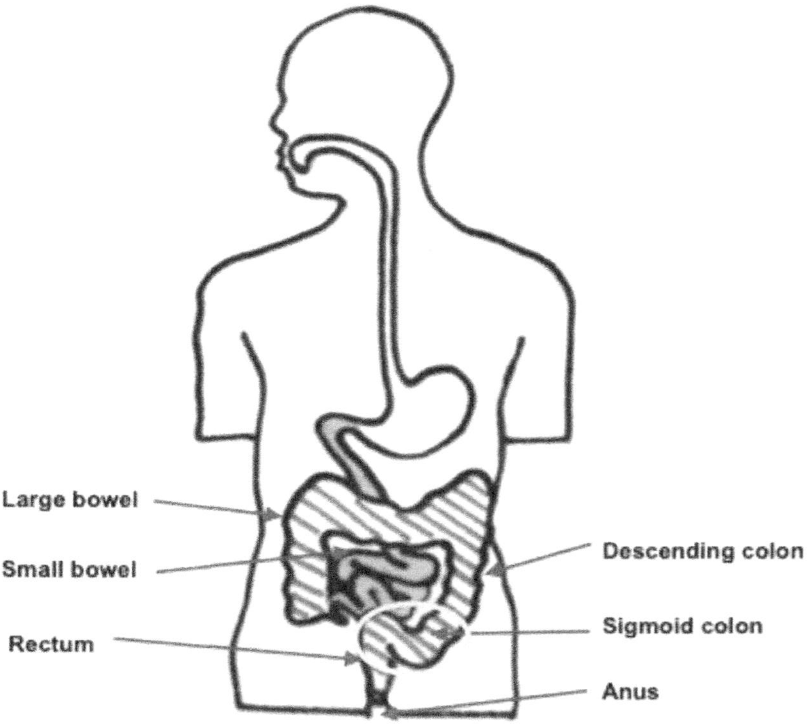

Waste left over from digested food is stored in the sigmoid colon until it is expelled through the rectum and anus. Figure 4 depicts an enlargement of the sigmoid colon area shown within the light blue ellipse above.

Figure 3: The gut (bowel) - small intestine, large intestine and rectum.

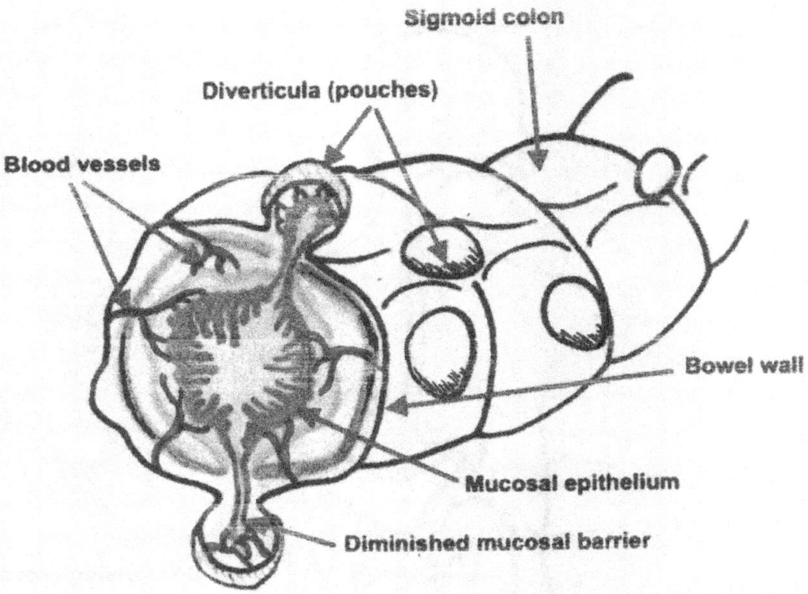

Gut permeability: the blood vessels in abnormal weak pouches could provide pathways for colonic bacteria and/or fungi to enter the blood stream.

Figure 4: Damage (diverticula) in bowel wall caused by constipation

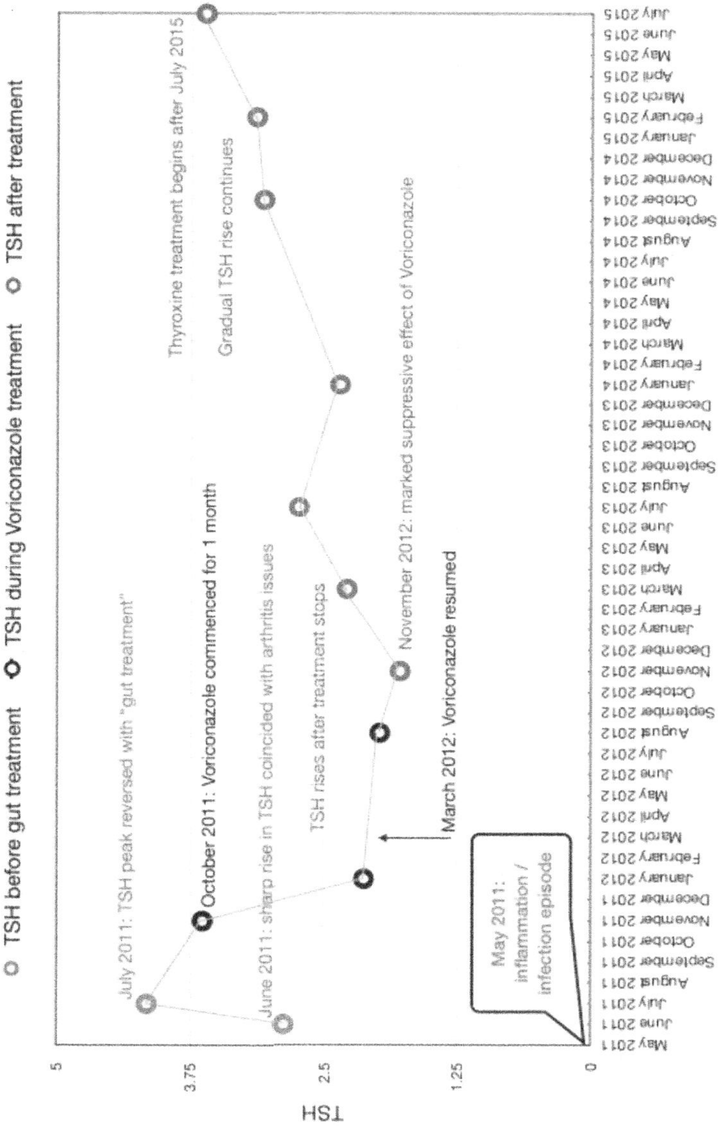

Figure 5: Thyroid function tests showing the effect of treatments

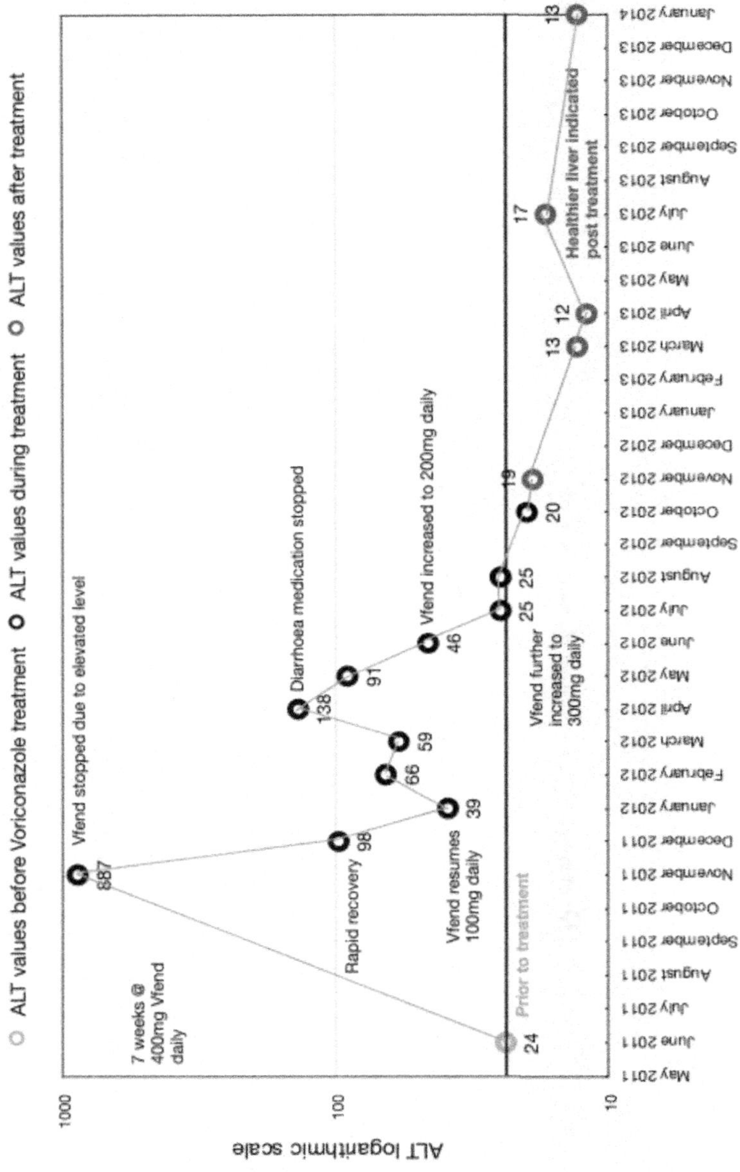

Figure 6: Liver function tests showing the benefits of Voriconazole

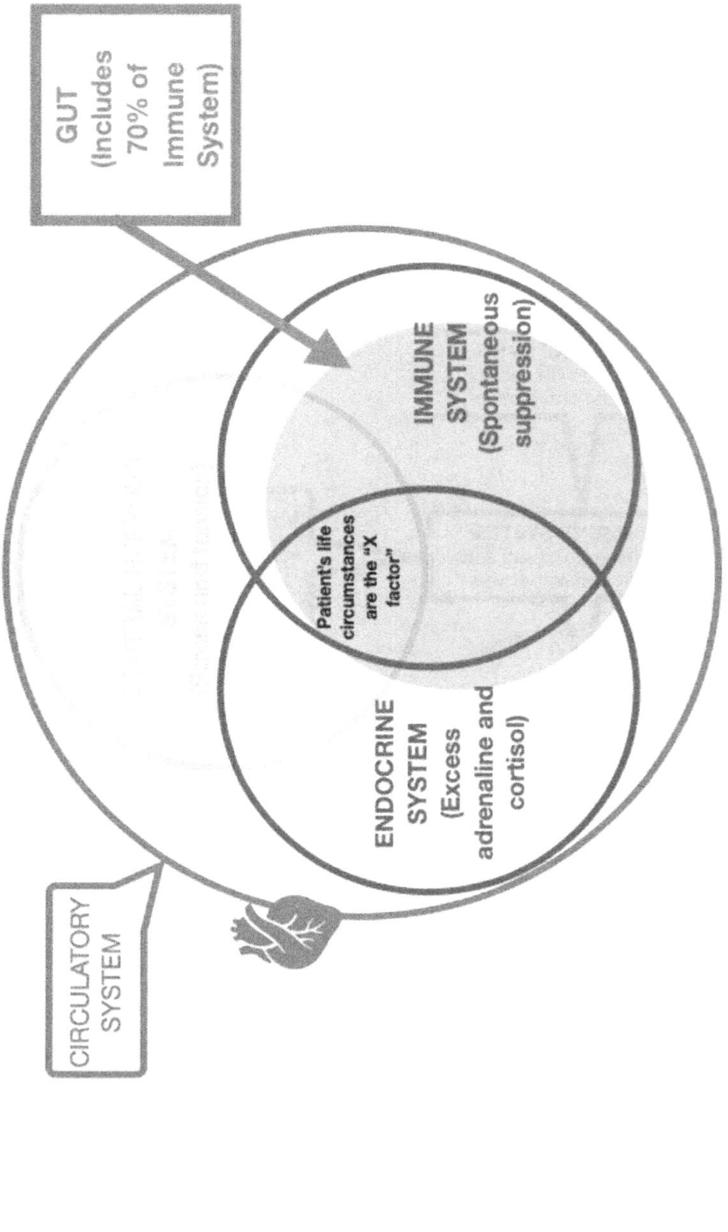

Figure 7: A lowered immune response caused by a patient's circumstances

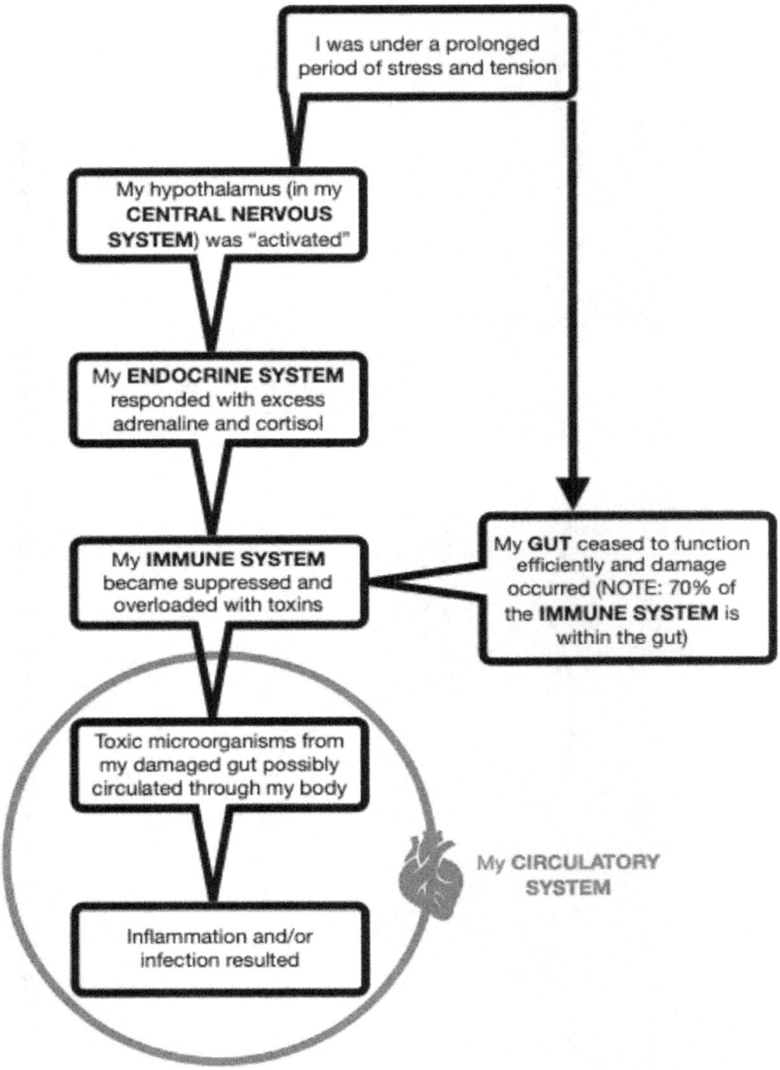

Figure 8: *My Concept* - chain of events resulting in inflammation and/or infection

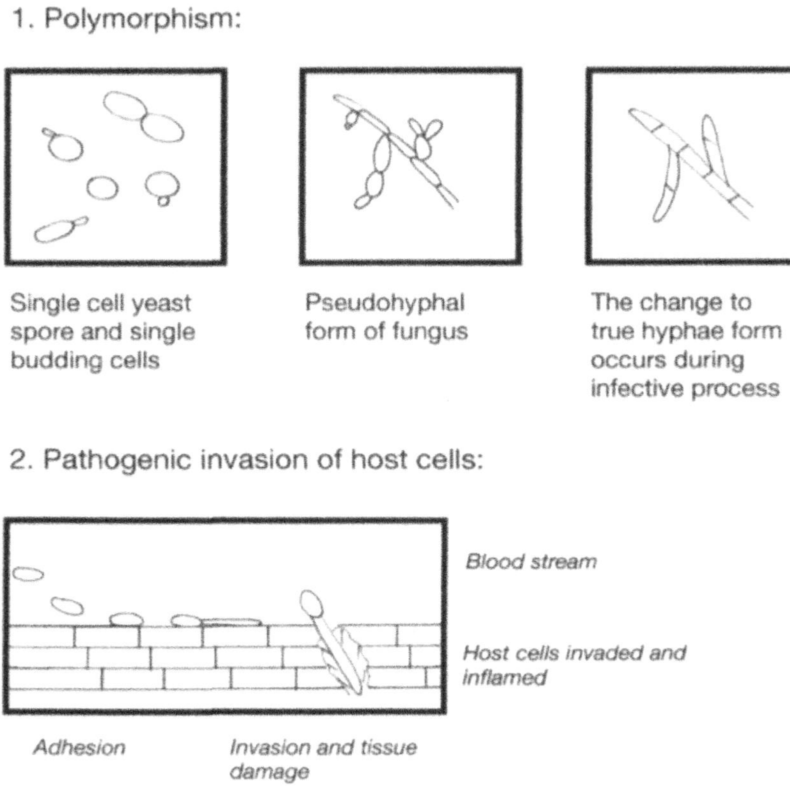

During infection process, *Candida albicans* quickly morphs into a hypha. Polymorphic adaptability enables it to infect almost any organ via the blood stream.

Figure 9: Malignant capabilities of Candida albicans

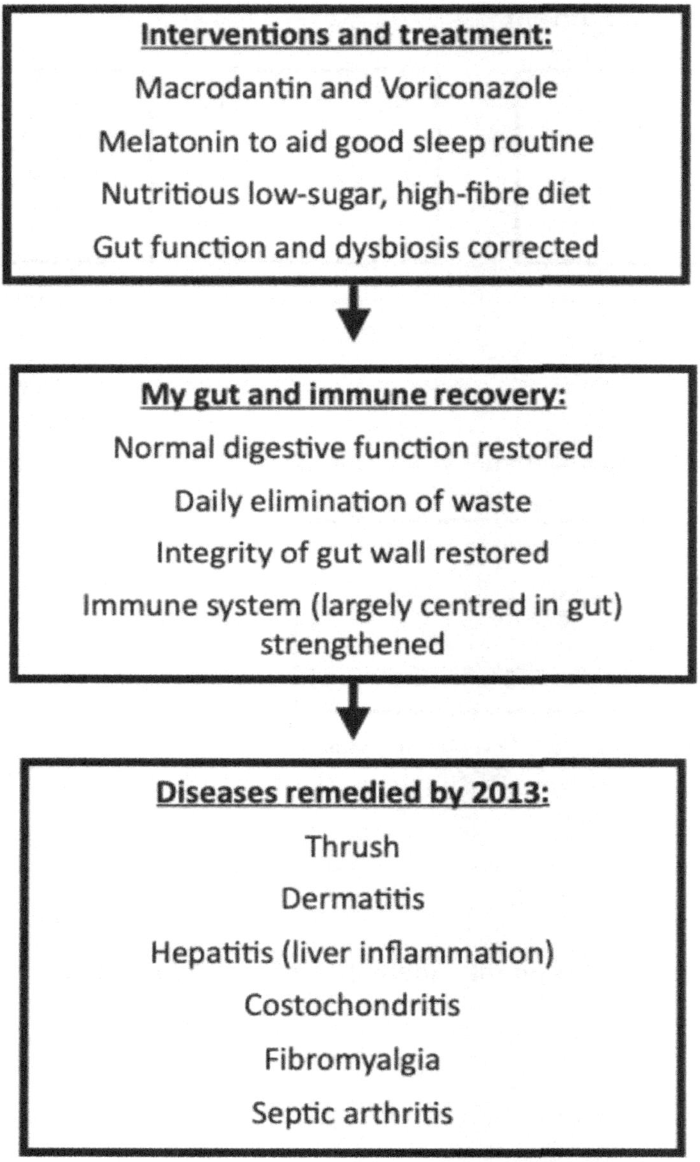

Figure 10 : Diseases treated with gut health interventions, antibiotics and antifungals

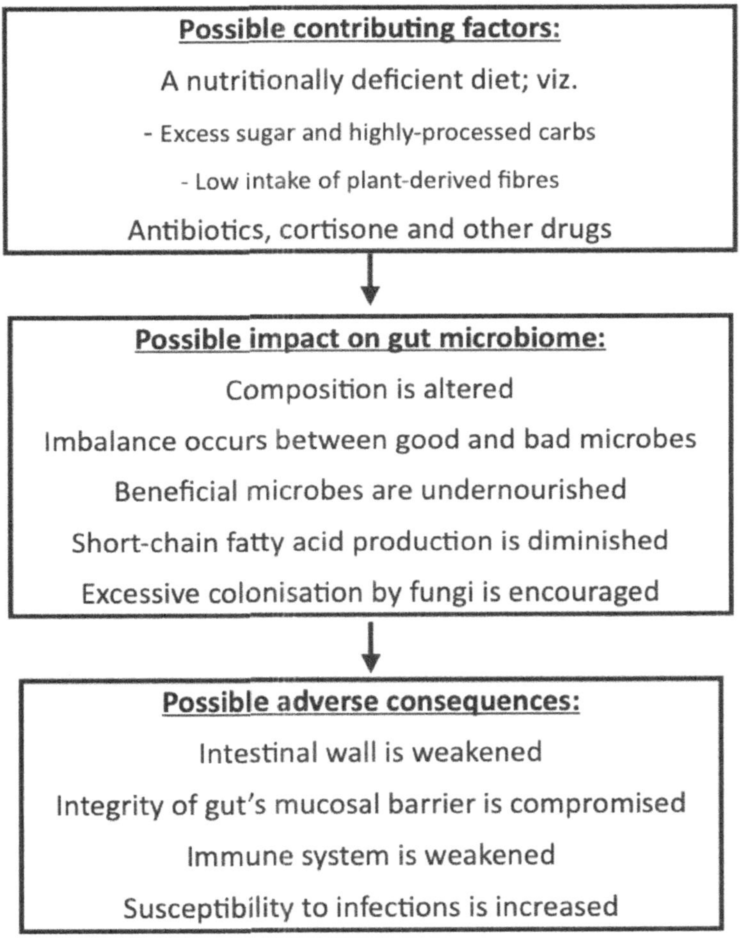

Figure 11: Dysbiosis/microbial imbalance in gut

Possible contributing factors:

Stress / Tension:

Constipation; bowel damage.

Unhealthy diet:

Fungal overgrowth enabled; beneficial microbes in gut undernourished; fermentation of insoluble fibres reduced; production of acids (such as acetate & butyrate) diminished.

↓

Possible adverse consequences:

Diverticulosis (pockets in bowel wall) develops

Waste matter collects and putrefies

Gut's mucosal barrier compromised

Intestinal lining becomes permeable

Immune cells in gut wall weakened

Immune system debilitated

↓

Possible impact on joints:

Pathogens enter bloodstream

Wave of pathogens unchecked by immune system

Blood stream disperses infective microbes

Toxic microorganisms embedded in joints

Inflammation occurs and cysts arise in joint cartilage

Erosion ("wear and tear") in joints initiated

Figure 12: My Concept - a theoretical understanding of my arthritis and the gut connection

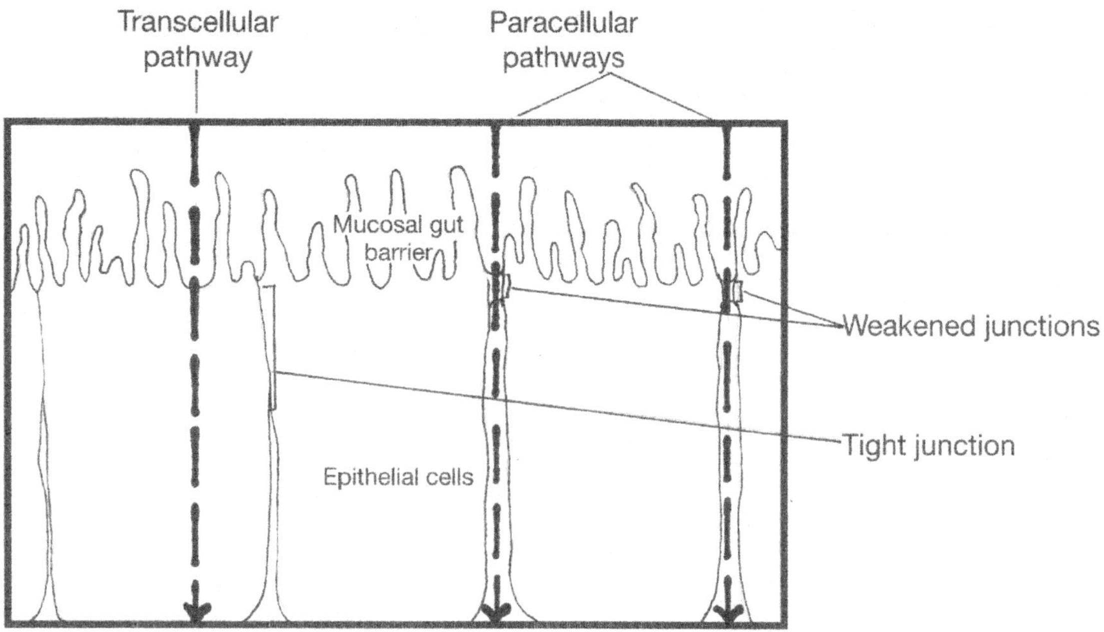

Intact tight junctions normally regulate microscopic pathways. When weakened by chronic constipation gut permeability can occur.

Figure 13: Translocation pathways through gut barrier

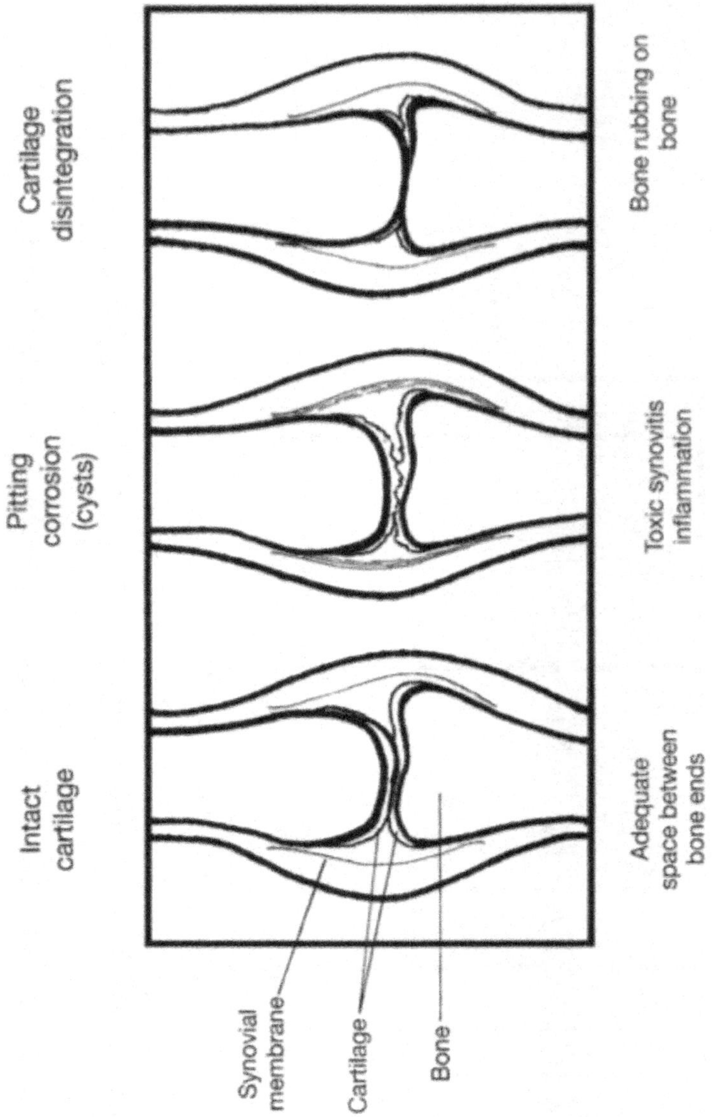

Figure 14: Cartilage disintegration initiated by infective toxic synovitis

Appendix B GLOSSARY

Acetabulum: the socket of the hip bone, into which the head of the femur fits

Acupuncture: a component of traditional Chinese medicine where fine needles are inserted to release stress-relieving endorphins

Adaptive immune system (acquired immune system): a subsystem of specialised immune cells and antibodies that eliminate pathogens or prevent their growth; adaptive immunity is created in response to exposure to foreign invaders

Aetiological agent: an infectious pathogen that causes disease

Alimentary canal: digestive tract; i.e. passage food passes through from mouth to anus during digestion

Allopathic Medicine: a term used to define science-based, modern medicine

ALT: an enzyme that is concentrated primarily in the liver; high levels indicate liver damage

Ankylosing Spondylitis: a form of spinal arthritis that affects the vertebrae; overtime the bones can fuse making the spine less flexible

Antigenic material (Toxins): substances the immune system doesn't recognise and tries to fight off by producing antibodies; an invading microbe (pathogen) is called an antigen that triggers the immune response; foreign molecules (components of a virus, bacterium, or parasite)

Antioxidant: a substance such as vitamin C that inhibits damaging free radicals

Autoimmune disease: "Friendly fire" occurs; i.e. a confused immune system attacks a part of our body

Biological system: a biological unit within the body consisting of organs that work together to carry out a particular task

Biomedical model: an approach that focuses on the physical or biological aspects of disease and illness; the medical model of care used in conventional medicine

BM: bowel movement; i.e. the discharge of faeces/excrement through the anus

BMD test: a bone mineral density test

BMJ: a weekly peer-reviewed British Medical Journal; a journal that champions research

Bowel: medical term for last 3 parts of digestive system; i.e. small intestine, large intestine and rectum

Butyrate: a short-chain fatty acid that has a powerful effect on gut and wider health

CAM: complementary and alternative medicine

Candida albicans: a polymorphic fungus that's a normal part of the healthy microbiota in the GI tract; harmless in humans with healthy immune systems

Candidemia: the presence of *Candida* yeasts in the blood; amongst the most common bloodstream infection of any kind

Candidosis (Candidiasis): a fungal infection typically on mucous membranes, caused by Candida species

Central Nervous system (CNS): the brain and spinal cord (the peripheral nervous system includes all peripheral nerves throughout the whole body)

Chondrocytes: cartilage-forming cells that maintain the cartilaginous matrix

Circulatory system: an organ system (also called cardiovascular system) that contains the heart and blood vessels; enables blood to circulate throughout the body

Colon: large intestine between small intestine (small bowel) and anus

Commensal parasite: a parasitic organism that causes no harm to the host

Costochondritis: an inflammation of the cartilage that connects the ribs to the breastbone

CSF: Cerebrospinal fluid

CSIRO: The Commonwealth Scientific and Industrial Research Organisation, Australia's national science agency

Cutaneous lesions: skin damage; e.g. eczema patches, spots, fissures or cracks

Dermatitis: a general term that describes a skin irritation

Dermatologist: medical specialist who treats skin disorders

Digestive system: organs that break down food into substances the body can use

Digestive tract: all parts of the digestive system; i.e. mouth (1st part) to anus (last part)

Dimples of Venus: medical term for a pair of harmless indentations on lower back just above the buttocks; a common anatomical feature

Diverticula: bulging pouches that can form in the lining of the large colon

Diverticulitis: inflammation and infection of diverticula

Diverticulosis: the presence of small pouches (diverticula) in large colon

Dr Thomas McPherson Brown (1906 – 1989): a rheumatologist who believed RA could be cured with antibiotics

Dry-needling: a technique to release tension in taut and knotted muscles, where fine needles use strong stimulation at trigger points / sometimes known as medical acupuncture

Dysbiosis: an imbalance between good and bad types of organisms in the gut; reduction in beneficial butyrate-producing bacteria

EBV: Epstein-Barr virus; one of the most common human viruses

"Elderly" label: a clinical practice guideline (ageist approach) that defines patients according to chronological age; an inappropriate term that can suggest frailty

Endocrine system: the glands and organs that release hormones into the bloodstream; hormones are carried to tissues and organs all over the body

Endocrine system's major hormone producing glands: hypothalamus, pineal body, adrenals, pituitary, thyroid & parathyroids, ovaries, testes

Endocrinologist: medical specialist who treats disorders of the endocrine glands

Endogenous infection: an infection caused by an internal source; e.g. a parasitic microorganism that is present in the GI tract &/or genital tract

Epithelial barrier: intestinal lining that prevents pathogenic bacteria from entering the body, while allowing essential nutrient absorption

Epithelium: thin outer layer of a person's skin, as well as the thin inner lining of the alimentary canal

Faeces: left over waste from fully digested food

FDA: Food and Drug Administration in USA

Femur: the bone of the thigh, articulating at the hip and the knee

Fibromyalgia: a rheumatic condition characterised by stiffness and localised tenderness at specific points on the body

Fight-or-flight response: an acute stress response that prepares the body to fight or flee; adrenaline triggers the body's fight-or-flight response

Free radicals: highly chemically reactive, unstable molecules; cause cell damage and oxidative stress

Functional medicine: a healthcare approach that focuses on identifying and addressing the root cause of disease

Gait: a person's pattern of walking

Gastroenterologist: medical specialist who treats disorders of the stomach and intestines

GI lesions: microscopic tears that occur anywhere in the gut; usually asymptomatic

GI Tract: gastrointestinal tract consists of all the parts of the digestive system; i.e. long tube from mouth to anus

Ginkgo biloba: an extract of the leaves from the maidenhair tree that's native to China; believed to enhance blood circulation
Ginseng: a root extract from the ginseng plant; believed to have anti-oxidant and anti-inflammatory effects and may strengthen the immune system
Gut: non-medical term for last 3 parts of digestive system; i.e. small intestine, large intestine and rectum
Guts: animal entrails / fish guts (removed when a fish is gutted) / colloquial reference to internal parts of a person's belly (a person's bowels)
Haematogenous dissemination: spread through the bloodstream
Hashimoto's thyroiditis: an autoimmune disease that causes a problem with the thyroid gland
Hepatitis: inflammation of the liver caused by viruses, toxins, some medications or excessive alcohol consumption; rarely by bacteria
Holistic model: an approach that considers all the parts of something as a cohesive whole
Homeostasis: a healthy state maintained by the constant adjustment of biochemical and physiological pathways
Human commensal (parasite): a microbe that lives in or on its human host; e.g. a fungus uses food in the gut supplied by the human host
Hunter-gatherer diet: primitive diet of whole, fresh food; i.e. various meats, fish, vegetables, fruit, eggs, nuts, seeds and honey
Hypothalamus: part of the brain below the thalamus; controls temperature, hunger, thirst, circadian cycles; modulates endocrine system and stress
Hypothyroidism: abnormally low activity of the thyroid gland
Idiopathic condition: a disease which arises spontaneously or for which the cause is unknown
IM doctor: a qualified medical doctor who combines conventional western medicine with evidence-based natural therapies
Immune system: a complex network of cells, tissues, organs, and the substances they make; defends the body against infections

Infectious disease specialist: physician whose area of expertise is the treatment of infections

Inflammatory mediators: compounds that are either locally released or carried in blood or tissue fluids and may participate in initiating, perpetuating or aggravating a pathological process

Innate immune system: a defence system we're born with, that wards off bacterial and viral infections presenting at the mucosal cell surface; a first line of defence consisting of natural killer cells etc.

Integrative Medicine (IM): the blending of conventional medicine with evidence-based natural, complementary treatments and life-style interventions

Intestinal flora: Bacteria and other organisms that live inside the in-testines

Intestinal mucosal barrier: the epithelial barrier consisting of a mu-cosal layer as well as epithelial cells

***'it'*:** a medical condition that's not yet officially recognised by mod-ern, conventional medicine; a complex gut-related group of ailments where septic arthritis can be a late complication

Joint Aspiration: a procedure to remove fluid from the space around a joint using a needle and syringe

Kellgren-Lawrence Radiographic Scale: a 5 grade classification scheme of OA - no OA, doubtful, mild, moderate or severe; a clinical tool developed in England by rheumatologists Kellgren and Lawrence in 1957 for the radiographic diagnosis of OA

Leaky gut (increased intestinal permeability): a condition in which bacteria and toxins are able to "leak" through the intestinal wall; some mainstream doctors do not recognize the condition

Microbiologist: scientist whose area of expertise is the study of mi-croorganisms; e.g. bacteria, viruses, fungi, algae and some types of parasites

Microbiome (microbiota): vast army of microbes in the gut that break down food to release energy and produce vitamins

M-on-M hip replacement: a metal-on-metal hip implant with a co-balt and chromium femoral head and a metal acetabular cup

My Concept: my theory of a chain of events in the body that result in inflammation/infection and disease

Mycoplasma: a genus of bacteria; the mycoplasma species are the smallest bacterial cells yet discovered; parasitic bacteria that can lack cell walls and cause disease

Nervous system: consists of two subdivisions – the central nervous system (CNS) and the peripheral nervous system (PNS)

Nocebo effect: where a patient's condition worsens because of what they're told to expect

Nutrients: chemical compounds in foods essential to life and health

Osteoarthritis (OA): a disease where degeneration of joint cartilage and the underlying bone occurs

Osteopenia: a medical condition in which the protein and mineral content in bone tissue is reduced; less severe than osteoporosis

Osteoporosis: a medical condition in which the bones become brittle and fragile from a loss of calcium; typically results from a deficiency of oestrogen, calcium or vitamin D

Oxford Hip Score: a patient-reported questionnaire used to evaluate the physical condition (function and pain) of OA patients requiring hip replacement surgery; a score that reflects OA patients' physical function, developed in England in 1996

Paracellular transfer: the movement of substances across an epithelium by passing through the intercellular space between the cells

Paraesthesia: an abnormal tingling sensation caused by pressure on peripheral nerves

Pathogens: microscopic organisms/microbes that can cause disease; e.g. bacteria, viruses, fungi and toxins (chemicals produced by microbes)

Peristalsis: the involuntary contraction and relaxation of the muscles of the intestine; wave-like movement that pushes waste matter out of the GI tract

Physiotherapist: an allied health professional qualified to treat disease, injury, or deformity by physical methods such as massage, heat treatment, dry-needling and exercise

Placebo effect: where a person's health appears to improve with treatment that looks real but has no therapeutic effect; a positive response to 'dummy' treatment

Polymorphic fungus: an organism like *C. albicans* that can grow as yeasts, pseudohyphae or hyphae; can colonise mucosal surfaces, or cause superficial, deep-seated or systemic infections

Prebiotic: leftover non-digestible fibre in gut that promotes the growth of beneficial micro-organisms

Probiotic: a substance which stimulates the growth of beneficial intestinal flora

Probiozyme: a blend of dairy-free probiotics and digestive enzymes.

Prophylactic treatment: treatment given or action taken to prevent disease

Prophylaxis: a preventative treatment or action; e.g. a preoperative antibiotic

RA: rheumatoid arthritis is a progressive disease where inflammation in joints results in painful deformity and immobility

Range of motion/ROM: the capability of a joint to complete its full spectrum of movements

Reductive explanation: a basic reason presented in a simple, undeveloped, crude form; e.g. "wear and tear" not "post infection erosive arthritis"

Referred pain: pain felt in one part of the body that's caused by an injury or disease elsewhere

Rheumatologist: medical specialist who treats diseases of the joints, muscles and bones

Risk factors: contributing features that increase the likelihood of a disease developing

Septic Arthritis: an infection in the joint (synovial) fluid and joint tissues; the infection usually reaches the joint through the bloodstream

Sigmoid colon: short curve of colon/large intestine just before the rectum

Sternum: the breastbone that forms the central part of the chest wall

Stool: another medical term for faeces (includes undigested food, bacteria, mucus, cells from epithelium)

Systemic candidiasis: (Disemminated candidosis): an infection of two or more non-contiguous deep-organs following haematogenous spread

TCM: (see Traditional Chinese Medicine)

TGA: Therapeutic Goods Administration in Australia

THR: total hip replacement

Thrush (candidiasis): a vaginal yeast infection caused by the fungus *Candida*

Thyroiditis: inflammation of the thyroid gland

Thyroxine: the main hormone secreted into the bloodstream by the thyroid gland

Toxin: a poison especially one produced by or derived from microorganisms and acting as an antigen in the body

Traditional Chinese Medicine: a medical system that has been used for thousands of years to prevent, diagnose and treat disease. Treatments include acupuncture and herbal therapy.

Transcellular transfer: where substances pass through the epithelial cells, passing both the apical membrane and basolateral membrane

Transient candidemia: the temporary presence of *Candida* yeasts in the blood

Transient toxic synovitis of the hip: an inflammation and swelling of the tissues around the hip joint; a condition usually affecting only one hip that lasts a short time

TSH: Thyroid-stimulating hormone

Vfend: brand name for voriconazole, a medication used to treat fungal infections

WOMAC OA index (Western Ontario and McMaster Universities arthritis criteria): a set of standardised questionnaires used to evaluate the physical condition of OA patients; a tool that measures arthritic pain, stiffness and physical function developed in the USA in 1982

Yeast/*C. albicans* spore: a single-celled unit that's part of the fungi life cycle; spores adapted for dispersal and reproduction

Appendix C RESOURCES

BOOKS:

Arthritis Australia, 2013: Joint replacement, Arthritis Foundation, W.A.

Arthritis Australia, 2015: *Taking control of your osteoarthritis,* Indegene Publishers, Australia.

Arthritis Research UK, 2011: *Complementary and alternative medicine for arthritis,* Chesterfield, UK.

Australian Broadcasting Corporation, 2017: *Everything you ever wanted to know about osteoarthritis,* Radio National Health Report – Dr Norman Swan interviewing Professor David Hunter.

Beinfield, H. and Korngold, E., 1991: *Between heaven and earth. A guide to Chinese medicine,* Random House, New York, USA.

Bird, T. and others, 2018: *The CSIRO Healthy Gut Diet,* Macmillan Publishers, Sydney, Australia.

Brand-Miller, J. and others, 2002: *The new glucose revolution; to achieve weight loss, blood glucose control and life-long health with GI,* Hodder, Sydney, Australia.

Brownstein, D., 2001: *Overcoming arthritis,* Medical Alternatives Press, Michigan, USA.

Cahalan, S., 2013: *Brain on fire,* Simon & Schuster, New York, USA.

Campbell, G.W., 1972: *A doctor's proven new home cure for arthritis,* Harper Collins Publishers, London, UK.

Crook, W.G., 1986: *The yeast connection.* Random House, New York, USA.

Doidge, N., 2007: *The brain that changes itself; stories of personal triumph from the frontiers of brain science,* Penguin, New York, USA.

Doidge, N., 2015: *The brain's way of healing,* Viking Penguin, New York, USA.

Enders, G., 2014: *GUT; the inside story of our body's most underrated organ*, Scribe Publications, London, UK.

Gillespie, D., 2008: *Sweet Poison...why sugar makes us fat,* Penguin Books, Melbourne, Australia.

Greger, M., 2017: H*ow not to die; discover the foods scientifically proven to prevent and reverse disease,* Pan Macmillan, London, UK.

Heffernan, M., 2011: *Willful Blindness...why we ignore the obvious at our peril,* Walker Publishing, New York, USA.

Hitchcock, K., 2014: *"The medicine".* The Monthly, 14:April.

Hoare, J., 2019: *The woman who cracked the anxiety code,* Scribe Publications, Melbourne, Australia.

Jenkins, J., 2011: *Rheumatoid arthritis; a self-help guide to getting on with your life*, How To Books Ltd, Oxford, UK.

Jenner, C., 2011: *Arthritis; a practical guide to getting on with your life*, How To Books Ltd, Oxford, UK.

Lam, P and others, 2002: *Overcoming arthritis; a holistic plan to relieve pain and restore mobility*, Dorling Kindersley Pty Ltd, London, UK.

Lane, N.E. and others, 2002: *All about osteoarthritis; the definitive resource*, Oxford University Press, UK.

Luntz, S.,2012: *"Arthritis Pain is outside the Joints".* Australasian Science, 9:July/August.

Noakes, M. and others, 2005: *The CSIRO Total Wellbeing Diet*, Penguin, Melbourne, Australia.

Perlmutter, D. and Colman, C., 2004: *The better brain book,* Riverhead Books, New York, USA.

Peterson, J., 2018: *12 Rules for life; an antidote to chaos,* Penguin Random House, UK.

Phelps, K. and others, 2011: *General practice; the integrative approach,* Elsevier, Sydney, Australia.

Richardson, M.D. and Warnock, D.W., 2012: *Fungal Infection; diagnosis and management,* Wiley-Blackwell Publishers, Oxford, UK.

Ross, H.M., 1987: *Fighting depression,* Larchmont Books, Atlanta, USA.
Shilts, R., 1988: *And the band played on,* St. Martin's Griffin, New York, USA.
Singh, H., 1992: *The missing dimension in medicine; caring for the whole person,* Whole Health Institute conference paper, Perth, WA
Weatherby, C. and Gordin, L., 1999: *The Arthritis Bible,* Healing Arts Press, Rochester, USA.

WEBSITES:

Arthritis Foundation of Australia: **arthritisaustralia.com.au**
Arthritis Foundation USA: **www.arthritis.org**
Arthritis Foundation of Western Australia: **www.arthritiswa.org.au**
Arthritis Research UK: **www.arc.org.uk (2011-2016)**
Institute for Complementary and Natural Medicine:**www.icnm.org.uk**
Natural Therapists Association of Australia - ANTA:
www.australiannaturaltherapistsassociation.com.au

ABOUT THE AUTHOR

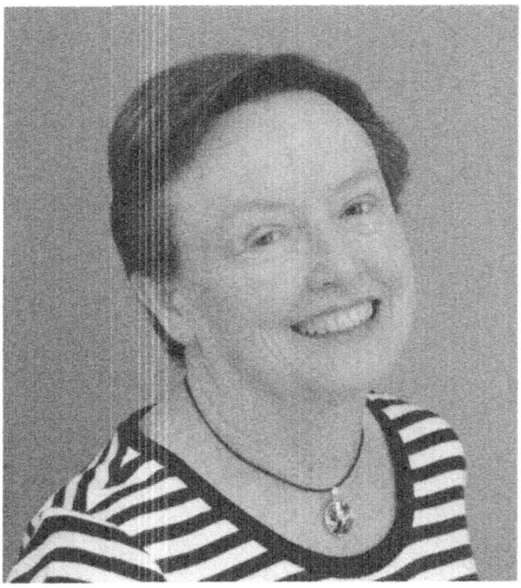

Mary Anne Lilly, author of *Arthritis and the gut connection*, began professional life as a secondary school teacher having completed a master's degree by research with distinction. Later in life she returned to university to study librarianship. Although born in South Africa, Mary Anne regards Perth, Western Australia as home where she's lived for most of her life. When not focused on her arthritis project, Mary-Anne delights in long walks and entertaining her five grandchildren. She's a believer in ageing well, remaining active, doing what one enjoys and not being a burden on one's children.

Made in United States
North Haven, CT
04 November 2026

21763960R00157